Ambulatory Care Systems

Volume II

Ambulatory Care Systems

Ambulatory Care Systems

Volume II
Location, Layout, and Information Systems
for Efficient Operations

Richard J. Giglio
University of Massachusetts

Lexington Books
D.C. Heath and Company
Lexington, Massachusetts
Toronto

Library of Congress Cataloging in Publication Data

Giglio, Richard J.
  Location, Layout, and information systems for efficient operations.

  (Ambulatory care systems ; v. 2)
  Includes index.
  1. Clinics—Location. 2. Clinics—Planning. 3. Clinics—Administration—
Data processing. I. Title. II. Series.
RA966.A46   vol. 2   362.1'2'08s [362.1'2]   76-55865
ISBN 0-669-01324-2

To Sally, Jennifer, and Lindsley

Contents

List of Figures

List of Tables

Preface

Providing ambulatory care is in many ways an odd sort of enterprise—at least from the viewpoint of a planner. Ambulatory care is expensive, and yet for the majority of clients it is difficult to measure or even describe in precise terms the product that is being produced. In fact, the *product* and the *client* are one and the same, which makes for a confusing situation at best. In those all too rare instances where it is possible to develop a rational structure for making a decision about the operation of a facility, so-called nonquantifiable or political considerations often cause one's beautiful plans to be twisted out of shape or abandoned altogether. Forecasting is difficult, and yet attempts to control the market by promotional means which are used in other fields are unacceptable.

Clients often come for service when they have no medical problems and stay away when they do. And despite ornery customers (or is it products?), irrational forces, and the inability to predict what will happen or even measure what did happen, nearly everyone agrees that outpatient services are important and that every community should have access to them.

In light of all the difficulties involved, it is not surprising that the planning and management of outpatient clinics are often called an "art"—certainly it is not a science. Many individuals have made heroic efforts to formulate and validate various types of planning models which would add precision to management decision making. These models are often complex, which makes them inaccessible or expensive and impractical for managers to understand and use. And the results of the models cannot be accepted at face value because they contain explicit and implicit assumptions which the practitioner must take into consideration. Thus a dichotomy exists: practitioners make decisions with relatively few quantitative aids while many sophisticated models sit on the shelf.

This book represents an attempt to bridge the gap between theory and practice. Because of the nature of this approach, the text runs the risk of being considered nonrigorous by theorists and/or not detailed enough by practitioners. However, the author hopes that by simplifying theoretical methodologies and providing detailed decision-making frameworks, the book will prove a useful adjunct to decision making.

This book represents part of the work of an interdisciplinary team of researchers at the University of Massachusetts, who have worked for the past six years on a project titled, "The Design and the Evaluation of Outpatient Systems," under the sponsorship of the National Center for Health Services Research, HRA, HEW, HS-00709. The senior investigators on this research team came from the fields of operations research, industrial engineering, public health, and sociology, and they have been assisted by health administrators, physicians, economists, and psychologists.

Much of this work has been reported piecemeal in over fifty papers, journal articles, presentations in national and international meetings, and in a series of short courses. The response we have received from these presentations, and the evidence we have obtained from our visits to ambulatory care centers across the country, indicates that a comprehensive design and evaluation manual is badly needed. We hope this set of volumes begins to fill this need.

Our research procedure has been to identify problem areas through conversations with people in the field, personal observation, and examination of the literature. The next step was to find a local facility that appeared to have such a problem and focus on that facility to help solve the problem; then we generalized our experiences as far as possible to develop a methodology that would benefit others in the same circumstances. If there were questions in our minds as to whether the techniques that were developed would work in other places, we would test them in another facility of a different type that had the same problem. Through this procedure, essentially a series of case studies set in perspective, we have developed these volumes. This procedure has not put us in contact with all the problems likely to arise in the course of designing (planning) and operating an outpatient facility; however, it has led us to most of the important and ubiquitous problems; and it has also assured us that the results growing from this work are practical and useful for today's outpatient facilities.

The titles for the volumes in this series are as follows:

Volume I   Design for Improved Patient Flow
          Edward J. Rising

Volume II Location, Layout, and Information Systems for Efficient Operations
          Richard J. Giglio

Volume III Evaluation of Outpatient Facilities
          Paula L. Stamps

Volume IV Designing Medical Services for Health Maintenance Organizations
          John R. Coleman and Frank C. Kaminsky

Volume V   Financial Design and Administration of Health Maintenance Organizations
          John R. Coleman and Frank C. Kaminsky

This volume of the series covers three aspects of planning and ambulatory care facilities:

Part I   How to choose a location for a facility
Part II How to plan a space layout for a facility
Part III How to design an information system for the facility

The topics were grouped in one volume because in setting up a facility the three tasks would have to be performed more or less in sequence. Although there are interrelations among the areas, each part of the book can be read separately with little loss of continuity.

In a continuing effort to update our material and keep our work relevant, we invite comments from the users of volumes in this series. In the past some of our most helpful comments have come from letters from those who have attended presentations we have made. We hope these volumes will also elicit a wide response, and a form to encourage this response has been inserted in the book. We are interested in not only the usefulness and relevance of the material but also what other areas or problems need examination.

Acknowledgments

This set of books is not the exclusive product of the authors themselves, but is the result of effort by a research team that at times numbered as many as ten people. This work was supported largely by the National Center for Health Services Research, HRA, HEW under the title, "The Design and Evaluation of Outpatient Systems," HS-00709. This division of the Health Resources Administration, under Gerald Rosenthal, has supported programs that will make available the newer technologies in a usable form for health and medical care facilities that need assistance; this series of books is a result of their policy. We would like to acknowledge especially the assistance of our project officers, Dirk Speas, Allen Berkowitz, and Wardell Lindsey, whose encouragement and attention to our needs has made it possible to do our best work.

The author wishes to acknowledge the following individuals who, although mentioned later in a general way, have had a special part in the development of the material presented in this book. Harpal Dhillon, Ph.D., carried out original research on facility location which was incorporated into Chapter 3. David Rumpf, Ph.D., contributed much of the work on physical layout. Eric Kyllonen, M.S., greatly extended and expanded some initial research of Lloyd Taylor, M.S., in developing procedures for planning information systems.

The author's thanks go to Philip Hertz of the Holyoke Health Center for his interest and patience in providing an initial site for the research and his insight and encouragement throughout this process. Special thanks go to Nancy B. Eddy who, as a researcher and administrator, assisted us with both the implementation of our work and the organization and presentation of our results.

This work would not have been possible without the help of a number of hospitals, outpatient facilities, medical clinics, and health centers which have cooperated with us by spending their time explaining problems, by permitting us to collect data, and by accepting our advice and allowing us to observe the consequences. These facilities, in effect, became our "laboratory." This has not always been easy for them, and we gratefully acknowledge their help and their progressive attitude.

Albany Medical School, Albany, NY

Amherst Medical Associates, Amherst, MA

Darnell Army Hospital, Killeen, TX

Harvard Community Health Plan, Brighton, MA

Holyoke Health Center, Holyoke, MA

Medical West, Chicopee, MA

Mercy Hospital, Springfield, MA

Ryder Hospital, Humaco, Puerto Rico

Springfield Hospital Medical Center, Springfield, MA

University Health Services, Amherst, MA

University of Massachusetts Medical School, Worcester, MA

Valley Health Plan, Amherst, MA

Worcester Hahnemann Hospital, Worcester, MA

We feel we must express our debt to the generations of graduate students at the University of Massachusetts who have worked on elements of this research as part of their theses, dissertations, and projects, as well as those students who were research assistants and worked under direct supervision. Many of these students have their names cited as authors and as coauthors of the journal articles, presentations, and reports that are referred to as source documents of this work. Because many of the others worked just as hard (or perhaps harder) on other topics on which less progress was possible, and therefore do not appear as authors in the references, we are listing alphabetically all the names of those who assisted as contributing researchers.

Donald Allen	Bryan Luce
Bob Baron	Theresa Morgan
Marcia Bondy	Dzung Nguyen
John Coleman	Faika Shannban Nour
Brandon Delaney	L. Brad Prenney
Harpal Dhillon	Stephen Roberts
Osman El-Refaie	David Rumpf
Suzanne Fields	Dina Slavitt
Edward Hannan	Lisa Sokol
John Kaminsky	Sandra Sturdivant
Eric Kyllonen	Lee Taylor
Oscar Lawson	Jack Watts
Murray Lebowitz	

We also owe considerable thanks to the secretaries and administrative assistants who, over the years, have assisted us with the research in ways too numerous to mention and typed our manuscripts in an uncomplaining way.

Jerrie Glazier	Ann Quigley
Deborah Hurwitz	Claude Shepard
Adrianne Kamsler	Linda Souza

Finally, thanks go to Phyllis Glazier for her assistance with the final manuscript, to Doris Connors for her uncomplaining secretarial help over several years, and to Nancy B. Eddy for editorial help, advice, and the supervision of the actual publication.

Amherst, Massachusetts   *Richard J. Giglio*
July 1977

Part I:
Planning the Location
of an Ambulatory
Care Facility

Introduction

Chapters 1, 2, and 3 of this book describe methodologies designed to help planners determine either the location of freestanding ambulatory care facilities or whether they should be constructed at all. Much of the material comes from journal articles on location planning. However, the chapters are not a review of the literature in the normal sense of the word, although reference is made to several articles. Rather, the data and methodologies reported in journals are used along with actual planning experiences to develop methodologies for ranking alternative locations for outpatient facilities.

First the importance of location planning is discussed along with the difficulties and problems inherent in trying to determine optimal locations in a scientific way. The different types of location-planning situations are described because, for example, an individual trying to determine a location for a federally supported clinic for a rural area faces a somewhat different set of problems than does an administrator planning a group practice in a suburb. Principles which apply to all location-planning situations are presented along with practical aspects common to most. Then the process (when, who) of planning is described for several environments. Planning methodologies are presented for each of several key planning situations. The methodology of Chapter 2 is practical and relatively easy to use and does not demand large amounts of data, although it can use data of nearly any level of sophistication which the planner has available or believes is appropriate to get. Chapter 3 contains a procedure for the regional planning of facilities. That procedure relies on an extensive data base and requires a computer program. The computer program is available through the National Technical Information Service [1], and guidance is provided for data collection in that publication. However, the users must decide whether they have the incentives, resources, and time to employ the more sophisticated decision-making aid.

The order of topics in this part of the book progresses from the most basic and general to the most sophisticated and specific. Thus, the reader can stop at any point of the section and still have information and calculations which can be helpful in evaluating alternative locations.

Reference

1. Harpal Dhillon and Richard J. Giglio, *A Computer Model for Planning Locations, Capacities and Schedules of Outpatient Facilities*, Report Number UMASS/IEOR-77/2 (Springfield, Va.: U.S. Dept. of Commerce, National Technical Information Service, 1977).

1

Background on Location Planning

Importance of and Difficulty of Location Studies

There is no doubt that the location of a facility affects the way clients will use its services. Both common sense and several studies attest to this fact. The importance of location relative to other factors depends on the particular situation. Closeness is often not the major consideration in a choice between facilities, and so often the location of a facility can be made on an intuitive basis. Conducting a scientific analysis to determine the optimal location of a facility is very difficult because of the multiplicity of factors which affect the perceived distance of a clinic: a facility can be close in distance but not in time or convenience if potential clients do not have a full range of transit alternatives; a facility can be psychologically distant if it is in a neighborhood which a client perceives as being different from his or her own. Social and cultural factors play a large role in the effective distance between a client and a facility, and these factors also are not easy to incorporate into formal decision-making aids. Therefore it is no surprise that many planners find the literature of location planning incomplete. Nevertheless, theoretical constructs and the experiences of others can be useful to any planner, especially if they are incorporated into a coherent methodology whose limitations are clearly understood.

The Literature of Location Planning

There is an extensive literature on location planning much of which is described in Chapter 3. A fair amount concerns the location of hospitals, a lesser amount concerns that of outpatient facilities. For many planners the literature will be confusing for a number of reasons: it often pertains to a particular facility; it is often very theoretical; frequently there are certain implicit assumptions which may not apply to the particular user.

A careful reading of the literature leads to some overall conclusions. Location affects which facility an individual will utilize more than it does the level of usage. Unfortunately, the effects of location on utilization are known only in general terms, and studies do not arrive at a consensus with regard to a quantitative description of the attractiveness of a facility as a function of distance. This is not surprising because the effects of distance depend upon the region and particular population involved. Geography is not the most important characteristic governing the use of facilities, and so studies of the effects of location can yield accurate descriptive models only if all other important factors are accounted for—a nearly impossible task. Indeed, it is unlikely that location decisions will ever resemble an exact scientific activity unless a nationwide health insurance program results in a set of homogeneous guidelines and facilities which probably would not fully serve the needs of the diverse American population anyhow.

Characteristics of Location Problems

The health care industry is extremely complex, and different groups in different settings can have widely divergent goals, although these goals often are not stated explicitly. Before the location of a facility is determined, it is crucial that the planners accurately and explicitly state their true objectives. To help in this task, a framework for representing the dimensions or differing characteristics of location-planning problems is described in the following paragraphs and summarized in Table 1-1.

Health care delivery is both a business, that is, an entrepreneurial activity, and a public, subsidized service. To admit to the former, as nearly any private or group practice must, does not imply insensitivity or the provision of poor care to clients. Rather it implies that the location chosen will be one that serves a population which can support the practice and that another, possibly more needy, segment of the population might not be served. On the other hand, a public decision-making body probably would choose to locate near the more needy population.

In planning location one must reflect on who is making the decision and who will underwrite the costs of conducting the analysis. A small private practice simply does not have the time or resources for an extensive study. A health maintenance organization (HMO) would have more resources and a greater need to conduct location studies. A government group trying to meet needs in large underserved regions would have even more resources and incentive to collect data and conduct significant location studies. All planners, however, should limit the scope and complexity of their studies to be consistent with the uncertainties and inaccuracies inherent in the location-planning process. There is no point in collecting large amounts of data and using sophisticated models to calculate predicted utilizations to the second decimal place when inaccuracies in the data and a lack of knowledge about why individuals choose particular facilities make it very difficult to predict demand or need with even a 10 percent accuracy.

Is one planning an individual facility or a network of several clinics to satisfy a regional demand? The latter situations argue for a detailed location analysis while in the former instance choosing the location on the basis of judgment alone can be a reasonable approach.

Table 1-1
Dimensions of Location Problems

	Type of Analytic Techniques				
	Based on Demand	Based on Need	Based on Capacity to Support	Analytical Model Used	Model Based Only on Judgment and Experience
Entrepreneurial vs.	A	N	A	O	O
service objectives	S	A	O	O	S
Private vs.	A	S	A	O	O
government	O	O	O	O	S
Individual facilities vs.			A	S	O
areawide			O	O	O
Specific location vs.			O	S	O
general location			O	O	S
Adquately served vs.	A	N	A		
underserved	O	A	O		
Ample time vs.				O	O
short time				S	O
Data available vs.				O	S
little data				S	O

A = Almost always
O = Often
S = Seldom
N = Almost never

Is one trying to determine a general location, i.e., a town or area of a city, or is one trying to choose the exact location for a clinic? One set of factors pertaining to demand, need, and/or a population's capacity to support a facility should guide the choice of a general location while the choice of specific location will be influenced most heavily by practical aspects such as zoning, traffic patterns, availability of parking, and, of course, property costs.

Different models apply for medically underserved and adequately served areas. For underserved areas, the facility should be located so as to be accessible to the largest number of people; but if there are other facilities in the area, "competition" from those facilities has to be taken into account.

In an entrepreneurial situation the economic considerations usually play a major role. In other instances the objectives to be met by choosing a particular location are not as obvious. Some objectives which have been suggested are (1) proximity, e.g., within 30 minutes travel time for the residents of a geographical area, (2) maximum utilization, and (3) minimal distance for those who use the facility. Although the above objectives are related, researchers [2] have shown that they can lead to widely differing choices of location. Thus precision in stating objectives is required.

The availability of data inevitably exerts a strong influence on the type of analysis which is feasible. If data are readily available and accessible, for example from a health systems agency (HSA) the costs of making an analysis are much less than if the data have to be obtained through sampling. Similarly, time pressures have a strong influence on the type of analysis which would be cost-beneficial. Decisions which have to be made almost immediately simply do not lend themselves to reflective, methodical analyses.

The dimensions of location problems are schematically represented in Table 1-1 along with the characteristics of the most appropriate analytic techniques. The analytic techniques are categorized according to whether they are predominately analytic or judgmental and whether they strive to meet demand or need. This categorization will be also followed in succeeding chapters. Reference to this table should help a planner pinpoint his or her particular problem and choose the most appropriate analytic aids.

Practical Considerations in Location Decisions

There are a number of practical considerations which are of paramount importance in choosing the location of ambulatory care facilities. Although most of these may appear obvious, there are innumerable instances where one or more have been ignored or overlooked with unfortunate results. A list of these factors follows:

1. Cost of renovation or construction at a particular site. This is perhaps the most obvious—and most important—of the "practical considerations." For new construction, the condition of the site and the availability of utilities and services are of paramount importance; for an existing building the costs of renovation have to be estimated—a task which takes some skill. However, an architect or engineer can usually determine the relative costs of building in competing locations. Be sure to allow for overruns in evaluating architects' estimates, especially if the construction might be deferred 6 months or more. The architect can supply you with the *Engineering News Record* construction index [3] which helps you estimate inflationary effects.

2. Zoning. Before investing much time in studying location, check on zoning regulations. It is not uncommon for medical facilities to receive a variance if they are nonconforming, especially if medical services are in short supply.

3. Space available for future additions to the facility if expansion is contem-

plated. Population projections which are needed to evaluate alternative locations can indicate whether or not expansion is likely.

4. The preferences and objections of interest groups. As is discussed in Chapter 2, planners must anticipate community reactions. This is usually best handled by having representatives of those groups on the planning body.

5. Wishes of the staff. It is relatively easy to assess the preferences of an existing staff. They should be asked to rank competing sites and to indicate those to which they have particularly strong objections. In the situation where new staff must be hired, the planners must use their subjective evaluation to rule out specific locations which will make hiring particularly difficult. It is sometimes difficult to recruit staff for medically underserved areas. However, the specific location within a general underserved area can be chosen carefully to be the most attractive to them.

6. Security. Both patients and staff need to feel safe from danger when going to or from a facility. Also, the choice of location will affect the likelihood of a break-in for drugs or money.

7. Parking. Ample parking must be provided, even for inner-city clinics. The section on space planning provides guidelines for parking space.

Some General Principles of Clinic Location

In addition to the practical aspects of planning location, there are a number of principles and some background information which a planner will find useful. Much of this information is used in the methodology described in the following chapter, but it can also help guide planners even if they use more subjective procedures to evaluate different sites for a facility.

It is generally accepted that a population base of 8000 to 10,000 is required to support a freestanding facility with two physicians. If the facility is linked to a hospital or if physician extenders are used, then a base of 4000 to 6000 should be sufficient [4]. If the primary goal is to provide care, with financial solvency being secondary, these estimates may not be of great interest. However, in most situations financial considerations are important, and catchment areas must be designed so both the density of clients and their distance from the facility will be consistent with the above figures.

Both common sense and a number of empirical studies indicate that distance is a barrier to the utilization of health services. Distance affects choice of a facility more than it affects overall utilization, but both effects have been documented. For example, one study [5] in a metropolitan area found that only about 10 percent of the population utilized the physician closest to them, but that same study indicated that 90 percent of the sample population used a physician from within a 7-mile or 30-minute radius. For HMOs, the situation is different. Once an individual is committed to a plan, she or he tends to choose the closest facility 70 to 80 percent of the time [6]. This undoubtedly is because the service at each of the HMO clinics is designed to be uniform, and they have been sited to compete with one another geographically as little as possible.

Some individuals are affected more than others by distance, in particular the old and the poor. In fact, although the poor generally need more health services, some groups use them less. Also, it is not distance per se which affects utilization. It is the difficulty and expense of access which is most conveniently measured in terms of time. Although time and distance can be expected to be correlated (although one investigator found they are not [5]), the two measures are not interchangeable and time is the more critical determinant. Therefore, knowledge of the client population's transit alternatives is necessary to develop realistic location plans.

As a rough rule of thumb, one can assume that in an urban area where medical facilities are available, the average client will travel 3 miles or 15 minutes to see a physician. Within this radius, distance is probably not the most critical factor in the choice of a facility. Past habits, rapport with physicians, the hours of operation of the facility, and social-psychological reasons influence clients more than distance—unless there is a facility within a short walk (that is, 5 minutes). Very few clients will choose a facility more than 7 or 8 miles or 30 minutes away if reasonable alternatives exist. Thus, in an urban or dense suburban area with "competing" health care facilities, one can roughly characterize patients as coming from one of three zones. The first is the immediate neighborhood where convenience is the overriding factor. Most clients will come from the second zone—1 to 7 miles, 5 to 30 minutes—and distance will be an important, but not major, factor in choosing a physician. Very few clients will come from beyond the second zone, and those who do have strong reasons which compel them to ignore the barrier of distance.

The same general pattern holds for facilities in rural and lightly populated areas except that the effect of distance is diminished because people are accustomed to traveling longer distances. There are no major studies available to provide definitive quantitative evidence concerning the effects of distance in rural areas. However, planners who have given a great deal of thought and study to facility location in rural areas have concluded that to be at all effective, facilities should be no farther than 15 miles from potential patients. Alternatively, a patient should be able to reach a clinic in no more than 30 minutes, even under adverse weather conditions. This implies that patients will have automobiles, and if they do not, it is nearly impossible to serve them using a conventional approach.

Aesthetic, psychological, and physical characteristics of one location versus another must be taken into account. This is best done subjectively although a simple questionnaire or even informal conversations might give clues to any strong preferences or aversions individuals had for a certain site. If they rely on questionnaires, planners should be aware of the difficulties in interpreting responses and not assume that people will do what they said they would. The subject of questionnaire design is too complex to discuss in this book but a planner should at least be aware of possible pitfalls. In brief, people will tend to answer questions as if their decisions were made on the basis of orderly, rational analysis which conforms to the values of their peers or to the values they perceive in the questionnaire. In fact, their behavior is more complex and may not appear rational to the analyst.

A clinic, and its site, must appear professional and competent if patients are to have confidence in it. On the other hand, it should not intimidate them by being pretentious. Thus the ideal location is one which is somewhat better, and more affluent-looking, or more prestigious than the neighborhoods which contain most of the clients. This principle must be examined critically because ideology also affects the desirability of a location. Some client groups may feel strongly that the clinic should completely reflect their neighborhood—at least for a while.

The location of a facility is only one component of a broader influence, *accessibility*, which encompasses appointment delay time, waiting time, hours when the facility is open, services offered by the facility, and physician-patient relationships. Accessibility is, in turn, only one of the factors which influence utilization. One writer [7] describes other factors as (1) predisposing factors such as knowledge of the existence of available health services and attitudes toward health services and physicians, (2) enabling factors such as income and health insurance, and (3) health status factors which can be measured by careful and often expensive surveys (e.g., disability days, sickness days, etc.). Because of the complex of factors which affect usage, it is probably unrealistic to try to single out location as an important variable and to develop complex models; such models may give the appearance of precision but will probably miss or misrepresent many important relationships. The methodology described in Chapter 2 was developed with the above caveat in mind because it is to be used to rank locations relative to one another with the understanding that only geographical considerations were considered. The geographical ranking is then used in conjunction with other information.

Before the methodology is discussed, it is instructive to examine the reasons for particular location selections in sixteen studies [4]. These studies are not representative in a scientific sense, but they offer a sampling of the types of reasons and analysis which usually guide location decisions. The numbers in Table 1-2 total more than sixteen because some decisions had multiple reasons.

We note that subjective analyses by physicians and planners are, in practice, the most important factors. Convenience to medical resources is also important. There is a conscious effort to serve medically deficient areas, but only in three instances were in-depth analyses performed.

Table 1-2
Reasons Influencing Location Decision of Sixteen Facilities

Analysis	Number of Times Used
Recognized need by	
Physicians	4
Planners or community leaders	5
Survey	3
Convenience of supervision, close to medical school, etc.	4
Serve specific underserved region	5
Sophisticated analysis taking many factors into account	3
Use existing facility	1

References

1. Harpal Dhillon and Richard J. Giglio, *A Computer Model for Planning Locations, Capacities and Schedules of Outpatient Facilities*, Report Number UMASS/IEOR-77/2 (Springfield, Va.: U.S. Dept. of Commerce, National Technical Information Service, 1977).

2. William J. Abernathy and John G. Hershey, "A Spatial-Allocation Model for Regional Health Services Planning," *Operations Research* 20 (3), 1972.

3. "Quarterly Cost Round-up: Building Cost Index for 22 Cities," published quarterly in *Engineering News Record* by McGraw Hill, New York.

4. Social Systems Research Corporation, *Methodology for Determining Optimum Sites for Placement of Free-Standing Ambulatory Care Facilities in Rural Maine*, Report Number HRP-0003865/3GA (Springfield, Va.: U.S. Dept. of Commerce, National Technical Information Service, 1975).

5. G.W. Shanon, J.L. Skinner, and R.L. Bashshur, "Time and Distance: The Journey for Medical Care," *International Journal of Health Services* 3 (2): 237-43, 1973.

6. J.E. Weiss, M.R. Greenlick, and J.F. Jones, "Determinants of Medical Care Utilization: The Impact of Spatial Factors," *Inquiry* 8: 50, December 1971.

7. P.F. Gross, "Urban Health Disorders, Spatial Analysis and the Economics of Health Facility Location," paper presented at the National Conference of Operations Research Society of America, October 1971.

2   A Planning Methodology

The Planning Process

It is crucial to distinguish between the process of planning and the analytic methodology used. The former concerns "who" and "when" while the latter deals with "how." Whatever methodology is used to analyze data and evaluate alternative sites, a sound process must be employed to permit the maximum input of knowledge and preferences.

Circumstances are too varied to suggest one type of decision-making process. However, it is possible to state some guiding principles.

The decision-making team and leader should be clearly defined.

State your objectives. Avoid hidden agenda items.

The separate tasks should be defined.

The time for analysis should be defined. A bar chart is a convenient tool to keep track of tasks and their schedule.

Formal provision should be made to solicit opinions, attitudes, and preferences from staff.

The attitudes and desires of potential clients should be sought in an open and well-defined manner. Before including specific client representatives in a decision-making or even advisory capacity, be sure you are aware of the consequences of their not agreeing with the staff's desires. Do not include community representatives "for show."

Study as many different alternatives as time permits.

Seek the help of HSAs, other clinics, and experts in any nearby universities. Very often someone else will have collected needed information or a part of the analysis can be used as a graduate student project.

Methodology

The methodology presented in this chapter does not require sophisticated computing machinery; a hand calculator will suffice. Also, using the method-

13

ology does not require a great deal of data. Population data available from the Bureau of Census are sufficient. If, however, data have been gathered by an organization such as HSA or if there are resources for extensive surveys, the more refined data can be used to yield more accurate results.

At the outset we must state that the methodology assumes that decision making occurs in an ordered, predictable world. In practice, some professional or community groups may have veto power or may influence location decisions for reasons which are difficult to include in a quantitative procedure and which may not appear rational from some points of view. Therefore, the methodology should be used to rank alternatives. The final location will be chosen from the ranked list on the basis of the so-called nonquantifiable factors.

Provided the objectives of the facility are known, the general framework provided by the methodology can be used for any problem. In some situations a particular step will be deemphasized or omitted altogether. For example, all situations require an assessment of need and demand although an entrepreneurial planner would have to stress the latter; planners must always consider competing facilities although there will be few in a medically underserved area; financial enabling factors are less important to a government-financed clinic while transportation enabling factors are likely to be more critical; all planners must deal with predisposing factors.

The general steps in the proposed methodology are outlined below and then described in greater detail along with specifications of the required data, some exemplary data, and a discussion of potential data sources. The steps in the analytic procedure are as follows:

1. Define service areas which are geographical clusters of the population.
2. Determine relevant population strata along with predisposing factors and enabling factors.
3. Estimate current and projected need for each stratum.
4. Estimate current and projected demand for each stratum.
5. Describe existing facilities and ambulatory care services and prepare a distance table and a timetable.
6. Evaluate alternative locations by determining their shares of total need and/or demand.
7. Review rankings with advisory group.

The methodology may be used at two levels—one general, the other specific—and often will be used at both levels for the same planning problem. It can be used to determine the county, city, or broad geographic area in which to locate a facility. This would be the case if a federal or state agency wished to find the most needy areas in which to place a clinic. Alternatively, a group of private physicians may wish to evaluate which of several regions holds the greatest promise for a practice.

The methodology can also be used to evaluate specific locations once the general area or town has been chosen. In many instances, planners will already have selected a general area and could use the methodology to pick the particular neighborhood. In other instances, the methodology would be used only to choose the general region with the particular location to be chosen on the basis of political or social considerations. The major difference between the two forms of analysis lies in the size and detail of the population groupings.

Define Service Areas

For a general location problem, service areas are most conveniently defined as *census tracts*. Typically, a census tract contains 4000 to 7000 people. For a more specific location problem, tract data may be useful, but service areas based on blocks or block groups will probably be more useful (except in rural areas). A census tract usually consists of 3- to 9-block groups.

Appendix 2A describes the census data and how it can be obtained. Of particular use in learning about available data is *A Data Acquisition and Analysis Handbook for Health Planners* [1]. In many instances, the regional planning groups such as HSA may have the required data. Often municipalities or hospitals also have these data available, so a quick inquiry may save the time and cost of getting the data from the census bureau. Title XV of the National Health Planning and Resource Development Act of 1974 (P.L. 93-641) mandates state health systems agencies (HSAs) to focus attention upon six factors. Each HSA must "assemble and analyze" the following:

1. Status (and determinants) of the health of the residents of its health service area—prevalence and incidence rates can be used to define "status" while measures of relative and attributable risks can help to describe "determinants."
2. Status of the health care delivery system and its use by residents.
3. Effect the area's health care delivery system has on the health of residents—prevalence and incidence rates measured over time and at different levels and quality of service help to measure effectiveness.
4. Number, type, and location of resources.
5. Patterns of utilization by residents.
6. Environmental and occupational exposure factors affecting the immediate and long-run health of residents.

Thus, HSAs should be willing and able to provide data for location studies.

Determine Relevant Population Strata

Census data describe populations in terms of age, sex, race, and economic and social status. All these characteristics affect usage, but for the methodology not all are of equal interest. Only those characteristics which most significantly affect utilization will be considered in the basic methodology described in this chapter. At the end of the chapter, however, we describe how a larger number of stratifications could improve the accuracy of precision at the cost of extra analysis. The major strata are sex, age (under 17, 17 to 44, 45 to 64, over 64), and ability to pay. Secondary strata are level of education (less than 8 years, 8 to 12 years, more than 12 years), income, and race (white and nonwhite). The effect of most of the secondary characteristics is uncertain. Not long ago, the poor made fewer visits to physicians, but nationwide this is no longer true. It is ability to pay rather than income which determines usage, and with health insurance and Medicaid more poor people now have the economic means to pay for care than ever before. However, many people of moderate means do alter their usage because of cost. High education tends to lead to higher usage, but again these results are mixed. It is difficult to untangle race effects from income effects, so no firm guidelines are presented in this book. However, if knowledge of local conditions (for example, data gathered by an HSA) demonstrates the way in which income, education, or race affects utilization, this knowledge can easily be incorporated into the analytic procedure.

The numbers of people in each stratum should be determined for the coming year and estimated for a point 5 years in the future. Planners can apply the growth rates of the general area to all the service areas. However, if one service area is expected to grow especially fast, such an effect should be noted.

Estimate Current and Projected Need

Generally, one thinks of a "need" in the population which, by enabling and predisposing factors, becomes a "demand." This construct makes sense from an intellectual point of view. However, "need" is difficult or even impossible to estimate. Need depends upon arbitrary norms. One person may feel he needs medical care when he has a cold, another may not. As the health system improves, its very competence generates new "needs" which were not perceived as needs earlier. Thus, from a practical point of view, the process of calculating demands by first determining needs is not very workable.

It is relatively easy to determine historical demand from statistical data; one must only count the numbers of people who sought medical care when it was available. Thus, one way to determine need is to infer it from demand. For a particular stratum, one can calculate what the demand would be if a facility were available. This will be called *apparent need*.

Estimates of demand can be based on *Current Estimates from the Health Interview Survey* [2], published by the National Center for Health Statistics. Using 1975 data with the major stratifications of age and sex, one can predict the following demand rates (Table 2-1). These data have some limitations—in

Table 2-1
Visits per Year for Population Strata

	Under 17	17 to 44	45 to 64	Over 64
Male	4.5	3.5	4.9	6.4
Female	4.0	6.2	6.1	6.8

particular, they document only visits to a physician rather than visits for services in an outpatient facility. Therefore, additional estimates have to be made if other services are to play an important role in the facility. For each potential service area, the numbers in each stratum should be multiplied by the visits per year to get estimated need expressed in terms of total visits per year. This should be done for current population estimates and for the 5-year projection.

Estimate Current and Projected Demand

Since *need* is being defined as expected demand under "average" circumstances, the projections already developed for each stratum in each service area can serve as demand in many circumstances. However, to reflect demand more accurately, enabling and predisposing factors should be taken into account. Some individuals in a service area may not have the financial means to pay for care because they are not eligible for Medicare but have income levels near the poverty line. Their visitation values should be reduced by 20 to 40 percent. Individuals with more than 12 years of education should have their rates increased by 10 percent. Any other local trends which are known can also be used to adjust potential demand.

Prepare Distance Tables and Timetables

List each existing facility along with the services if offers in a table. Also mark their location on a map. The table should show times between service areas and services offered. Travel times cannot be obtained by simply multiplying distance by an average rate unless the entire region is homogeneous—all suburban, all rural, or all urban. Walking speed can be estimated to be 2 miles per hour; for automobiles, expressway speed averages 50 miles per hour, rural driving speed 35 miles per hour, suburban 25 miles per hour, and urban 10 miles per hour.

Unfortunately, determining travel times is not always as simple as dividing distance by average speed for two reasons: some individuals will use mass transit, which involves a wait, and some individuals may not perceive distances accurately.

To determine the travel time for a stratum which does not use automobiles, the average travel time on the bus or subway can be estimated by simply measuring it. To the one-way travel time must be added an average wait which can be approximated by one-half the frequency of service or by 15 minutes, whichever is less. For example, if a subway to the facility runs every 20 minutes, a wait of 10 minutes would be added to the travel time. On the other hand, if the potential client is served by a bus which runs hourly, a waiting time of 15 minutes should be added to the one-way travel time. If public transit service runs less frequently than hourly, it probably is not a reasonable travel alternative.

For many reasons, often a person does not perceive distances, or travel time, in a mathematically accurate way. For example, if a person in a rural area is accustomed to traveling 10 miles to a town for shopping and other activities, that 10 miles most likely will not seem as far as 10 miles in another direction. It is possible to use a questionnaire on a sample of the population to estimate perceived travel times. Questions would be phrased so the respondent would choose between several overlapping pairs of locations on the basis of convenience so that relative perceived travel times could be calculated. The only other way to account for the effect of perceived travel times is to subjectively modify calculated times. Travel times to an area known to serve as a shopping or work center for a stratum of clients can be decreased by an amount, say 10 percent. On the other hand, travel times to an area seldom visited by individuals could be increased by 10 to 20 percent. The figures of 10 or 20 percent reflect some experience in a particular locale but should not be considered scientifically derived on the basis of a large sample of data. Therefore, planners should not hesitate to modify travel times according to their own perceptions.

Evaluate Potential Sites

The table of existing sites should be expanded to include travel times from each potential site or sites for the new facilities. Actually a series of tables should be prepared. Each table would contain the travel times for the existing facilities and the travel times for one of the new, alternative locations.

For each table the maximum geographical potential should be calculated. This maximum assumes that individuals will switch from an existing facility if a new one is significantly more convenient. Since patients tend to stick with existing providers of care, the answer will be optimistic from the standpoint of the new facility, hence the term *maximum* geographic potential. An emergency room which provides outpatient care with long waiting times would be less competitive with a new facility than would a well-run clinic which provides continuity of care. On the other hand, the vagaries of insurance sometimes make outpatient care in an emergency service economically more attractive to a patient. Therefore, we suggest that planners can adjust the geographic potential by use of a "loyalty" factor. A loyalty factor of 1 implies an average facility. A factor of greater than 1 implies clients are more likely to be more loyal to a particular facility. Thus, a clinic designed to provide ambulatory care may have a loyalty factor of 1.2 while an emergency room may have a factor of 0.8. These factors are what is known euphemistically as "educated guesses," but they do provide a way to include knowledge of nonlocation effects in the calculation of the geographic potential.

The analytic methodology assumes facilities will attract patients proportional to their geographical attraction, which is defined as the inverse of travel time. This attraction is modified by the loyalty factor described above.

The calculation can best be demonstrated by means of an example. Suppose there are 484 females aged 17 to 44 in service area 1. From Table 2-1 we can estimate that they will make 3000 visits per year for outpatient care. Also assume that this stratum is 10 minutes from facility A, 18 minutes from the new facility B, 22 minutes from C, and 30 minutes from D. Furthermore assume all facilities provide appropriate services for females, i.e., general practice and/or OB Gyn. Then the geographical attractions are shown in Table 2-2.

The maximum geographical potential of facility B of the stratum, females in service area 1, is

$$\frac{0.055}{0.643} \times 3000 = 257 \text{ visits/year}$$

The adjusted geographical potential of facility B of that stratum would equal

$$\frac{0.07}{0.56} \times 3000 = 375 \text{ visits/year}$$

To obtain the total geographical potential of a location, one need only sum the potentials of all the individual strata. An example is given in Table 2-3.

Table 2-2
Geographical Attractions of Competing Facilities

Facility	Attraction = Inverse of Travel Time	Loyalty Factor	Adjusted Attraction
A	1/10 = 0.1	1.0	0.1
B	1/18 = 0.055	1.2	0.07
C	1/22 = 0.455	0.8	0.36
D	1/30 = 0.033	0.9	0.03
Total attraction	0.643		0.56

Table 2-3
Sample Table of Expected Visits per Year

Service Area 1		
	Females under 17	287
	17 - 44	257
	45 - 65	375
	over 65	528
	Total females	1,447
	Males under 17	293
	17 - 44	112
	45 - 65	280
	over 65	528
	Total males	1,213
	Total from Service Area 1	2,660
Service Area 2		•••
	Females	•••
•••		
•••		•••
•••		
	Grand Total	82,128

Although the estimated visits per year for each location will be approximate, the rankings of different alternatives should be reasonably accurate. Estimates for each location were made using the same assumptions, so that if the geographic potential of one site is twice that of another, the planner can be sure that, from a geographical point of view, the former is a superior location. This quantitative information is valuable in considering other factors (cost, staff preferences, closeness to hospitals) which bear on location.

The breakdown of visits by service area and stratum is also very useful. It shows what types of individuals are most likely to come and, therefore, what services are most likely to be used. Also, once a facility has been opened, administrators can refer to the estimates, determine whether they are meeting their geographical potential, and see which service areas and strata are not using the facility or are using it to an unexpected degree. Such an analysis provides clues to the adequacy of existing operating procedures and may lead to changes such as educational programs designed to inform the public of services available.

Using the Methodology

It is clear that the above method was based on many compromises and represents only one way to bring some analytical rigor into the process of siting health facilities. Consequently, the methodology should never be masqueraded as the rigorous and scientific way to make siting decisions. On the other hand, the fact the methodology does not include many critical aspects pertaining to a facility's location should not be used to dismiss it as useless. When used properly, the procedures form an excellent base or starting point for the decision-making process.

Siting decisions should be a team effort involving medical staff, administrators, and clients. All participants in that process can understand the assumptions and limitations of the analytic method. The results of analysis provide a structure or focal point for discussion. For example, an individual who disagrees with the projections can refer to the analysis to say why. For example, national utilization rates may be too high and not applicable to the local situation; a competing emergency room may provide more competition than the model predicts because patients seem to like the service and the freedom to attend without having an appointment.

The analytic techniques described are quite rudimentary. In particular, utilization levels are based on only age and sex. For any area, census data exist which can be used to relate the income and education of individuals in a location to utilization rates [1, p. 109, vol. 2]. In addition, census data can be used to identify particular populations at risk [1, p. 108, vol. 2]. This information could be incorporated into the analysis by using strata based on those factors in addition to age and sex provided planners strongly believed the situation was stable enough to warrant the extra effort for precision.

The next stage in quantitiative decision making is described in Chapter 3 which presents a more comprehensive and complex model. Although that model promises to deliver more, it makes more stringent demands on the user, and for many situations planners would decide correctly to use the more basic analysis just described.

References

1. Anthony Oreglia, Denise A. Klein, Lee A. Crandell, and Paul Duncan, *A Data Acquisition and Analysis Handbook for Health Planners*, Volumes 1 and 2, DHEW Publication No. (HRA) 77-14506,7 (Rockville, Md.: Division of Planning Methods and Technology, Bureau of Health Planning and Resources Development, Health Resources Administration, 1976).

2. U.S. Department of Health, Education and Welfare, *Current Estimates from the Health Interview Survey* (Rockville, Md.: Public Health Service, Health Resources Administration, 1977).

Appendix 2A

The major source of population and socioeconomic data for health planning purposes is the U.S. Census Bureau. Information is available from the census on the total population of geographic area with breakdowns by age, sex, and race. The Census Bureau information is available in a variety of forms and from a variety of sources. The basic source is the U.S. Bureau of the Census, Department of Commerce. Specific questions and requests for data should be directed to the Central Users' Service, Bureau of the Census, Suitland, Maryland, 20222.

For most health planners, complete census data for the area in which they are interested would be available in either of two places; first, the regional HSA; second, any U.S. government depository—generally any large university library or a major metropolitan library will be a government depository.

Depending upon the size of the planning area, different census reports will be pertinent. In general, the easiest book for health planners to use would probably be the volume published for each state. The reference for that volume is as follows: U.S. Bureau of the Census, Census of Population 1970, Volume 1, Characteristics of the Population, Part #, State. Sold by Superintendent of Documents, U.S. Government Printing Office, Washington, D.C., 20402, $9.25.

In addition, a separate publication is available for each standard metropolitan statistical areas (SMSAs).[a] There are 241 SMSAs, each of which contains at least one city with a population of 50,000 or more plus adjacent areas which are integrated with the central city.

Census tracts are small, relatively permanent areas into which large cities have been divided. They are designed to be relatively homogeneous in population characteristics, and the average census tract has a population of about 4000.

Census tracts may also be divided into block groups which are a combination of contiguous blocks with an average population of about 1000 and also into blocks which correspond roughly to city blocks, with an average population of 100.

Census data are available in either printed form or summary tapes. Summary tapes can be purchased directly from the Census Bureau at $70 per reel, and they have much more detailed data than do the printed reports. Unless the user has appropriate computer equipment and programs, the most economical way to use the summary tapes is by a summary tape processing center. Some HSAs do have such capability.

A summary of reports available from the U.S. Bureau of the Census can be found in Table 2A-1. Also, *A Data Acquisition and Analysis Handbook for*

---

aCensus tract (*Location*), U.S. Department of Commerce, Social and Economic Statistics Administration, Bureau of the Census, PHC (1)-(*Number indicating location*). On sale by Superintendent of Documents, U.S. Government Printing Office, Washington, D.C., 20402.

Table 2A-1
Select Reports, 1970 Census of Population and Housing

Series PC(1)–A (one per state)	*Number of Inhabitants.* Final official population counts are presented for states, counties, SMSAs, urbanized areas, minor civil divisions, census county divisions, all incorporated places, and unincorporated places of 1000 inhabitants or more.
Series PC(1)–B (one per state)	*General Population Characteristics.* Statistics on age, sex, race, marital status, and relationship to head of household are presented for states, counties, SMSAs, urbanized areas, minor civil divisions, census county divisions, and places of 1000 inhabitants or more.
Series PC(1)–C (one per state)	*General Social and Economic Characteristics.* These reports will focus on the population subjects collected on a sample basis. Each subject is shown for some of or all the following areas: States, counties, SMSAs, urbanized areas, and places of 2500 inhabitants or more.
Series HC(1)–A (one per state)	*General Characteristics for States, Cities, and Counties.* Statistics on 100 percent housing subjects are presented for states, counties, SMSAs, urbanized areas, and places of 1000 inhabitants or more.
Series HC(1)–B (one per state)	*Detailed Characteristics for States, Cities, and Counties.* These reports focus on the housing subject collected on a sample basis. Each subject is shown for some of or all the following areas: States, counties, SMSAs, urbanized areas, and places of 2500 inhabitants or more.
Series HC(3) (one per UA)	*Volume 3. Block Statistics.* One report for each urbanized area showing data for individual blocks on selected 100 percent housing and population subjects. The series also includes reports for the communities outside urbanized areas which have contracted with the Census Bureau to provide block statistics from the 1970 census.
Series PHC(1) (one per SMSA)	*Census Tract Reports.* One report for each SMSA, showing data for most of the population and housing subjects included in the 1970 census. Some tables are based on the 100 percent data, others on the sample data.

Source: U.S. Bureau of the Census, The 1970 Census and You (Washington, D.C.: U.S. Government Printing Office, 1973), p. 7.

Health Planners, volumes 1 and 2 are very useful guides if one is anticipating using census data or making surveys. These handbooks are available from the Division of Planning Methods and Technology, Bureau of Health Planning and Resources Development, Health Resources Administration, Parklawn Building, Room 12-14, 5600 Fishers Lane, Rockville, Maryland, 20852.

3

A Quantitative Model for Planning Location, Capacities, and Operating Procedures

Introduction

This chapter presents a quantitative technique for planning the location, physical and operational characteristics, and scheduling rules for a set of outpatient facilities intended to meet the ambulatory health care demands of a defined population. The output generated by the model makes it possible to rank a number of alternatives in terms of predefined objectives. The best plan identified by this model can involve the augmentation of an existing set of facilities, the elimination of some of the existing facilities, or the establishment of a new set of facilities in a region having no existing facilities. The model is complex and requires a considerable amount of data. The mechanics of the model have been coded in FORTRAN, and copies of the program and running instructions are available through a federal depository [1].

Before the model is presented, it is appropriate to describe its function. It is desirable to plan facilities for ambulatory care on a regional basis so that all segments of a population have access to care. However, the implementation of such a policy presents many difficulties. First, there is the problem of defining *access* and determining how much an individual or society is willing to pay to make care more accessible. This aspect of the problem will be discussed in some depth.

Another problem centers on the organization necessary to do the planning and to see that it is implemented. Certainly, there is a general movement toward centralized planning. Although we can cite as evidence of better planning the activities of regional planning agencies such as HSAs and several studies which appeared in the literature [2, 3, 4, 5], it is not clear in all cases who would have the resources and authority to see that plans were made and followed. We do not address the question of planning agencies although we realize that the existence of a properly constituted planning agency is more important than the particular techniques used. Consequently, the usefulness of the model will depend upon progress made in the political sphere and the initiatives taken by health systems agencies (HSAs).

One final word of caution is in order: the problem is frightfully complex. Like many researchers who attempt to attack a realistic problem, we have seen our model and its concomitant data requirements grow to the stage where its size may discourage its use. We have tried to overcome this problem in two ways.

The author wishes to acknowledge Harpal Dhillon's substantial contribution to this chapter.

In one important area, empirical studies have been made in order to answer a question which will always arise in regional planning, to wit: How will a group of potential patients distribute themselves among a set of fixed facilities with a given spatial relationship [6] ?

The second way we tried to make the model more palatable was to structure it so that educated guesses could be used in place of hard data and so that segments of the model could be left out altogether without jeopardizing the algorithm used to find good solutions. The reader should bear this in mind while contemplating using the model on his or her problem.

A perusal of this chapter will give the reader a good picture of the types and form of much of the data necessary to locate facilities in a region in an optimal way. Unfortunately, we cannot provide data which would be applicable in individual situations because values vary by locale and they change over time due to inflation.

The Problem

In a given territory, the need for changing the availability of ambulatory health care may arise for several reasons.

1. The population of the area may grow.
2. There may be a shift in the population from some of the existing population centers to other centers in the planning region.
3. The perceived needs of the population may change.
4. Even without any significant changes in the population of various centers, changes in the economic, educational, and health status of the existing population can make it necessary to alter the existing system to provide primary health care more efficiently.

It is reasonable to attempt to design a system which satisfies demand while minimizing the sum of the investment and operating costs of facilities and the costs of travel and time of the clients who use the system. This objective is difficult to attain because there is no commonly accepted way to place a value on the patient's time and on the cost of her or his travel. Moreover, the demand on a system and the characteristics of that system are not independent. Demand on a facility is related to, among other things, the perceived travel time to the facility and the waiting time which a user has to spend in the facility before receiving service. The number of patients which a facility can handle also depends on the average waiting time allowed for a user, in addition to the facility's size and staffing. Consequently, the longer waiting times caused by an attempt to increase the throughput of a facility by leaving less slack in the appointment schedule may cause patients to seek their care from another provider. If there is any pretense of satisfying the preferences of the population, a planning model should take the above interrelationships into consideration.

Review of the Literature

There is substantial literature on both the behavior of clients faced with a choice of facilities and/or the methodologies which should be employed to plan a network of facilities to satisfy demand at a minimum cost. In the behavioral models, the so-called gravity concept of facility attractiveness has been most often adopted as the basic means for describing individual's choices of facilities [7]. These gravity models are based on the hypothesis that the attractiveness of a facility is inversely proportional to the distance between the residence of a user and the point where the facility is located [4]. A refinement of the gravity model is based on perceived travel time as a measure of the separation between the user and the facility [8, 2].

In dealing with outpatient facilities, there is an additional element involved in the estimation of facility attractiveness. This is the waiting time that a user spends in the facility before receiving the attention of a health care provider. This element of inconvenience has been considered in at least one study dealing with the location of primary health care facilities [5].

The attractiveness functions provide a basis for estimating the demand on each facility, and these estimates of demand are an essential element of all models for regional planning of service facilities. Coughlin [9] investigated the location efficiency of urban hospitals and physician offices as measured by patient and employee travel time. Schneider [10] developed statistical techniques for analyzing the location imbalance caused by the travel times associated within a given urban region. In 1965, Lubin, Drosness, and Wylie [7] used the "highway minimum path selection" technique for evaluating the existing and potential facility locations in a given planning area. Revelee and Swain [11] proposed one of the first models for optimal facility location in which cost was also considered. Toregas et al. [12] suggested a model for the location of emergency service facilities. In their model, there is an upper bound on the cost of building and operating the required facilities.

Abernathy and Hershey [2] proposed a planning model in which patient preference and socioeconomic strata are considered in addition to the distance to the facility sites. This is the first study which deals exclusively with the problem of facility location in a health maintenance organization (HMO). The HMO is treated as a unit, and the objective is to maximize the enrollment of patients for the entire HMO. This model can evaluate a finite number of sites, and all these sites have to be defined in advance. The location of a number of facilities at an equal number of predefined sites gives one possible configuration of the network of facilities. Each configuration must satisfy certain constraints including an upper bound on the total cost (fixed and variable cost of operating all the facilities) and a lower bound on the enrollment of each facility. The expected demand at each facility is estimated through the application of "attractiveness functions." Although the attractiveness function may indicate that the users at one population center will be distributed among many facilities, the model restricts the assignment of the entire population at one center to only one facility.

The requirement of predefined potential sites, assignment of the entire population at one center to one facility, and the lack of provision for considering the travel and waiting costs are obvious shortcomings in this model. The model presented in this chapter considers all major elements of cost and is capable of considering all feasible sites within the region.

Demand on Health Care Facilities

Whenever a number of facilities providing identical services are located at different points within a well-defined territory, they can be regarded as competitors, trying to secure the patronage of each individual within the area by providing maximum convenience in terms of accessibility and prompt service. This hypothesis concerning the relative attractiveness of facilities forms the basis of many investigations, several of which were described above. The mathematical formulation of this hypothesis leads to the development of "attractiveness functions" which will make it possible to estimate the extent of utilization of each facility within a given territory.

Convenience is probably not the major factor in a client's choice of facility. For example, habit and the personalities of physicians and nurses are important. However, a planner often has little control over these other variables; also they can be considered independent of the spatial distribution of facilities. If more were known about the attractiveness of a small "neighborhood" center relative to a larger and, as the folklore has it, less personal facility, this could be included in the model. However, the current lack of quantitative evidence has ruled out that possibility and left such decisions to the initiative of the planner or the political pull and tug of constituents.

A demand estimation technique based on the convenience of a facility was developed from empirical data and used in conjunction with the model. Space limitations prevent describing the technique in detail, but this omission does not detract from the description of the planning model which will work with any techniques for estimating demand. The interested reader is referred to Dhillon [6] and to a brief description included in the Appendix 3A. It should be noted that in the empirical study, the relative location of population centers and facilities only partly explained the way in which patients choose a facility. Consequently, from a statistical point of view, the parameters developed are not satisfactory. However, because of the inevitable number of confounding factors and all the personal considerations which affect choice of a physician or facility, we question the wisdom of trying models of ever-increasing complexity in an attempt to improve statistical significance.

Facilities and Population Centers

In the proposed model, the facilities represent the sources of primary health care, while each population center corresponds to an origin for the demand of health care. A network of routes connects various population centers with different facilities.

The location of each population center and facility can be expressed in terms of a set of coordinates, which also identify the location of any point in the planning region. In the absence of specific restrictions, every point in the planning region can be regarded as a potential site for the location of a proposed facility. However, some areas in the planning region may be ruled out of consideration as possible sites due to topographical restrictions, zoning restrictions, and other constraints. The proposed model has provisions for incorporating these location restrictions.

Distance Measurement and Perceived Travel Time

It has been observed that generally roads run roughly parallel to one another along two approximately perpendicular directions. This arrangement of the highway networks suggests that if the axes of reference are placed along the directions parallel to the general direction of roads, the highway distance between two points can be measured directly in terms of the coordinates of the two points. Referring to Figure 3-1, the distance between population center (PC) i and facility j, along the highway system, is given by

$$d_{ij} = \left[(|x_i - x_j|) + (|y_i - y_j|) \right] \times D$$

where D is the number of miles per coordinate unit.

The time for traveling from a PC to a facility is a function of the distance and the speed of travel. The speed of travel may be independent of the distance involved, or it may be a function of the distance. It has been observed that in some cases the perceived speed of travel increases with increasing distance up to a certain point [6].

The planner should try to observe the relationship between the distance traveled and the perceived speed of travel. If the nature of this relationship is known, the perceived travel time from any PC to any facility can be estimated

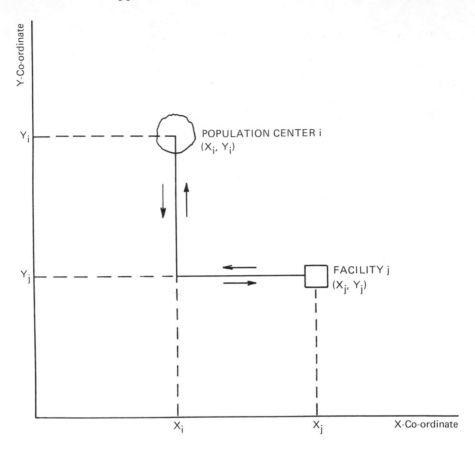

Figure 3-1. Assumed Path for Traveling from Population Center *i* to Facility *j*.

by identifying the coordinates of the two locations. In the survey which preceded the development of this model, this relationship was developed by correlating perceived travel times with the physical distance traveled by the respondents.

Facility Waiting Time and Facility Capacity

In order to get a good perception of the waiting time in a facility, it is necessary to study the queuing phenomenon which occurs inside a non-emergency health care facility. This queue can be analyzed as described in the text by Rising [13]. A summary follows.

1. A doctor's patients arrive at the facility at the appointed times, which are uniformly spaced in most cases. The interarrival time, for patients with

appointments, is usually fixed (constant). The nature of the interarrival time for walk-in patients can be ascertained by observation.[a]

2. The consultation time with a physician is a random variable, and Bailey [14] observed that the distribution of the consultation time X can be approximated by the gamma density function (Pearson Type III curve).

3. If there is more than one doctor in the facility and they are available for consultation at the same time, the queue usually does not differ in character from the situation when only one doctor is available. This is so because each user is assigned to a particular queue as soon as he or she enters the facility.[b] A user is not allowed to join the queue for a doctor with whom he does not have an appointment except for walk-in patients.

4. The average waiting time for a user depends on the difference between the interappointment interval and the average consultation time. The average waiting time can be kept short by having an interappointment interval significantly longer than the average consultation time. In the case of the queue of walk-in users, the average waiting time can be regulated by providing the number of queues necessary for keeping the average waiting time close to the desired figure.

5. Since the average consultation time cannot be altered significantly, the only means of reducing the average waiting time is to make the interappointment time longer. A longer interval between successive appointments will result in a smaller number of users per time period. Figure 3-2 shows the expected relationship between the average waiting time and the number of users served per time period for a facility. When the waiting time w_j is short, the number of user-visits which the facility can handle in a time period is small.

6. If the parameters of the distribution function for the consultation time can be estimated, the queue in the facility can be simulated. This would make it possible to estimate the average waiting time corresponding to a number of interappointment times. This estimation of the average waiting time can also be carried out through actual observation of the queue.

Facility Characteristics

Although standard designs are not very common at this time, most facilities share many characteristics, and it can be expected that centralized planning will

---

[a]Appointment patients arriving late are assumed to join the queue of walk-in patients. A missed appointment factor (a late arrival is also treated as a missed appointment) can be assigned to each facility. In the cost model, this factor can account for reduced health care provider utilization (appointment queues only) by increasing the service cost per user-visit. Patients arriving early are expected to wait until the time of appointment. No waiting cost is attributable to the waiting time prior to the time of appointment.

[b]This is the case when an appointment is made with a particular health care provider. If appointments are not made with specific doctors, but made for specific "times" only, the resultant queue would be classified as a "multiserver single waiting line" queue.

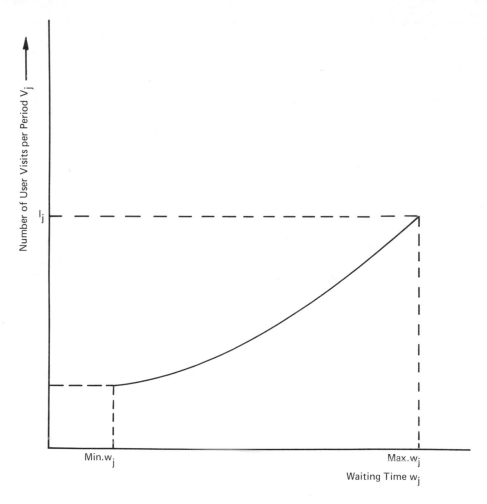

Figure 3-2. Expected Relationship between Number of User-Visits per Period and the Resulting Waiting Time.

further encourage the development of a few similar physical designs for outpatient facilities. In simplest terms, each facility design can correspond to a number of service channels within the facility. As an example, we will assume the existence of four categories of facility design, corresponding to facilities with 1, 2, 4, and 8 service channels respectively.

Among the benefits of a clinic shared by a number of doctors are better coverage for patients, savings in building cost, equipment cost, and in the wages of nonprofessional staff because of economies of scale. A facility with 8 service channels should have at least four times the capacity of one with 2 channels, but the building and equipment cost, and the cost of nonprofessional staff, will cost less than four times as much. Capital and personnel costs can be treated as "fixed costs" because the magnitude of these costs depends on the facility design class and is fairly insensitive to the number of actual users of the services of a facility.

Figure 3-3 shows the expected relationship between the maximum facility capacity l_j and the fixed cost per user-visit f_j.

Due to the restriction of the number of facility designs, it is evident that the maximum facility capacity cannot be increased continuously but takes place in steps. If a planner wants to have a maximum capacity different from the figure for a standard design, the fixed cost per period f_j will be that which applies to a facility design having a maximum capacity equal to or higher than the planned capacity.

For a given facility design class, there can be a range of values for the

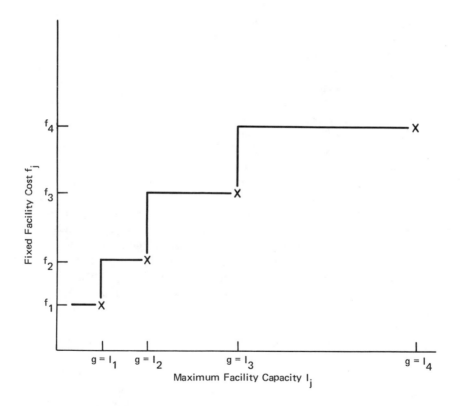

Figure 3-3. Discrete Nature of Fixed Facility Cost f_j as a Function of Facility Design Class g.

average waiting time. However, the interappointment intervals are generally restricted to three or four discrete values, for example, 10, 15, or 20 minutes. Corresponding to each interappointment interval there will be one value of average waiting time. Therefore, it is reasonable to include in the model a few discrete averages rather than let average waiting time vary continuously. The average waiting time for a facility can be identified by a waiting time class number. For any situation, waiting time is assumed to fall into one of approximately five classes. In the following discussion, the operational characteristic of a facility is identified by the waiting time class k. The example considered in Appendix 3A deals with a case in which four facility design classes are permissible for each facility design class, giving sixteen combinations of facility design and waiting time classes.

Total Facility Cost

In an outpatient facility, the cost per time period has two components: the fixed facility cost, which is relatively insensitive to the number of user-visits per period, and the operating cost.

In most outpatient facilities, the salaries of doctors and other professional staff constitute a major portion of the operating costs. Therefore, once the major characteristics of a facility are set, the fixed facility cost and the expenditure on staff salaries become invariable (if the staff is not paid on fee-for-service basis). The only variable element of the total facility cost per time period is the cost of supplies, which can be expected to be proportional to the actual number of user-visits per time period. However, this variable cost component amounts to a very small fraction of the total cost and can be ignored for location studies.

Although the total facility cost per period can be assumed to be constant for a given set of facility characteristics, the cost per user-visit depends on the number of visits. It is evident that for a given facility design class and waiting time, the cost per user-visit will be least when the facility is operating at its maximum capacity. This minimum cost is denoted by $q'_{k,g}$ where k is the waiting time class and g is the facility design class. If the number of user-visits per period is less than the maximum facility capacity $l_{k,g}$, the cost per user-visit will be higher than $q'_{k,g}$.

Figure 3-4 shows the expected relationship between the number of user-visits per period V_j and the total facility cost per user-visit Q_j for one design class and four classes of waiting time. These curves indicate that the maximum facility capacity increases as the average waiting time increases. For a given number of user-visits per period, the cost decreases as the average waiting time becomes longer.

Figure 3-5 displays the expected relationship between the number of

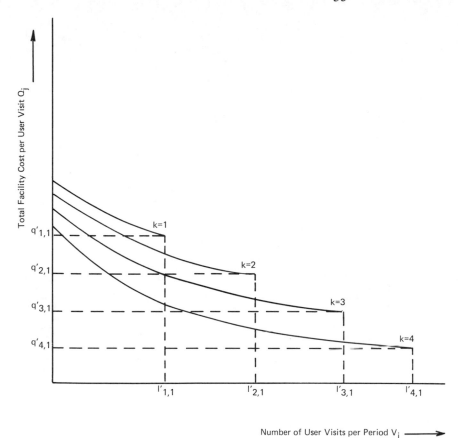

$q'_{k,g}$ is the minimum facility cost per user visit for a facility with waiting time class k and facility design class g. (1) In every case, the facility design class number is 1. (2) k represents the waiting time class number. (3) The maximum capacity of a facility with facility design class g and waiting time class k is represented by $l_{k,g}$.

Figure 3-4. Expected Relationship between the Number of User-Visits per Period and the Total Facility Cost per User-Visit for One Facility Design Class and Different Waiting Time Classes.

user-visits per period V_j, and the facility cost per user-visit Q_j for one waiting time class and four facility design classes. In this case, two features can be observed: for a given number of user-visits per period, it is most economical to have the smallest facility design class which can handle the demand; and, with a fixed waiting time, the minimum cost per user-visit occurs when the largest facility is being used at its maximum capacity.

Figures 3-4 and 3-5 suggest that the most practical method for estimating

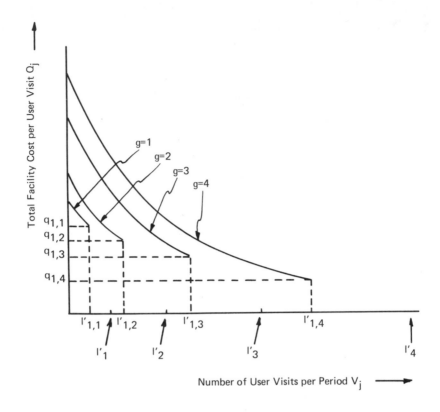

(1) In every case, the waiting time class number k is 1. (2) g is the facility design class number. (3) $l'_{k,g}$ represents the maximum facility capacity for a facility with design class g and waiting time class k. (4) l'_g represents the maximum facility capacity for a facility with design class g.

Figure 3-5. Expected Relationship between the Number of User-Visits per Period and the Facility Cost per User-Visit for One Waiting Time Class and Different Facility Design Classes.

the total facility cost per user-visit Q_j would be to determine the minimum total cost per user-visit for each combination of waiting time class and facility design class, and then estimate Q_j by relating the maximum facility capacity $l'_{k,g}$ (the minimum total facility cost per user-visit occurs when the number of user-visits per time period is $l'_{k,g}$) to the actual number of user-visits per time period V_j. Mathematically, this relationship can be expressed as follows:

$$Q = q_{k,g} \times \frac{l'_{k,g}}{V_j}$$

where $q'_{k,g}$ is the minimum total facility cost per user-visit for a facility with waiting time class k and design class g and j is the facility identification number.

Total Cost per Time Period for the Entire Community

The community of the residents of the planning region incurs the cost associated with the provision of primary health care. The total cost per period consists of three components: (1) cost of traveling to and from the facility; (2) cost of waiting inside the facility; and (3) total facility cost.

If T_i denotes the travel cost per minute for a resident of center i, the travel cost for a round trip to facility j will be equal to $2 \times (t_{i,j} \times T_i)$ where $t_{i,j}$ is perceived travel time from PC i to facility j. If W_i represents the waiting cost per minute, the waiting cost per user-trip to facility j will be equivalent to $(w_j \times W_i)$, where w_j is the average waiting time for facility j in minutes. The total facility cost incurred at facility j in one time period is given by $V_j \times Q_j$, where V_j is the number of user-visits and Q_j is the total facility cost per user-visit. The total cost per period for the entire community is given by

$$C = \sum_{j=1}^{n_0+n} \sum_{j=1}^{m_0+m} \left(U_{i,j} \times 2 \times t_{i,j} \times T_i + w_j \times W_i + \right) \sum_{j=1}^{n_0+n} V_j \times Q_j$$

where $U_{i,j}$ is the number of user-visits attracted to facility j from PC i, n_0 and n represent the number of existing the proposed facilities respectively, and m_0 and m represent the number of existing and proposed population centers respectively.

Optimization of the Cost Function

The objective of a health care systems planner is to provide either a required level of primary health care service at a minimum cost or the highest level of service for a given cost. The waiting cost per user-visit, as well as the inconvenience cost per user-visit, can be decreased by increasing the length of the interappointment interval. The lengthening of the interappointment interval causes a decrease in the number of user-visits per period, with a resultant increase in the total facility cost. Thus, an effort to decrease the inconvenience cost results in an increase in the total facility cost. In terms of facility capacity, an effort to attract more users (by reducing inconvenience) results in a reduction in the maximum facility capacity (because of a longer interappointment interval). The planner is confronted with the task of balancing these conflicting elements in an effort to optimize the utilization of resources.

The existing facilities can handle additional demand only to the extent of the difference between the total current demand and the total maximum capacity of all existing facilities. If the projected number of user visits exceeds $\sum_{j=1}^{n_0} l_j$, where l_j is the maximum capacity of facility j, additional facilities will be needed. However, the nature of additional demand could be such as to require additional facilities even though the projected demand is less than $\sum_{j=1}^{n_0} l_j$. Such a situation can arise when the proposed population centers are far from all existing facilities and also when the required changes in the operational characteristics of facilities result in unacceptably long waiting times.

In some cases, it will be possible to take care of the additional demand by changing the operational characteristics of the existing facilities, and it may not be desirable to build new facilities. However, the total cost of providing primary health care may be less when new facilities are planned. So planners should consider the possibility of setting up new facilities even though such facilities are not essential for meeting the increased demand.

Model for Evaluating Alternatives

For evaluating different alternatives, some of which may involve the setting up of new facilities, it is necessary to develop a model in which the coordinates of the n proposed facilities are decision variables, along with the design character-istics of the proposed facilities and the waiting time characteristics of all facilities. The number of new facilities n can also be regarded as a decision variable.

Mathematically, this model can be stated as follows:
Minimize

$$C = \sum_{j=1}^{n_0+n} \sum_{j=1}^{m_0+m} \left(U_{i,j} \times 2 \times t_{i,j} \times T_i + w_j \times W_i \right) + \sum_{j=1}^{n_0+n} V_j \times Q_j$$

subject to

(1) $h_{i,j} \geq 0$ for all i and all j ($h_{i,j}$ is the number of users going to facility j from PC i per period)

(2) $\sum_{j=1}^{n_0+n} h_{i,j} = h_i$ for each i (h_i is the number of potential facility users at PC i per period)

(3) $\sum_{i=1}^{m_0+m} U_{i,j} \leq l_j$ ($U_{i,j}$ is the number of user-visits attracted to facility j from PC i per period)

and facility design characteristics to remain unchanged for $j = 1, 2, \ldots, n_0$, and

(4) $\quad \displaystyle\sum_{i=1}^{m_0 + m} U_{i,j} \leqslant l_j \quad$ for $j = (n + 1), (n + 2), \ldots, (n_0 + n)$

In words, the objective is to minimize the total cost of service per time period, subject to these constraints: (1) no facility is overloaded, (2) the existing facilities remain at their current locations and their physical characteristics remain unaltered, and (3) the location of the new facilities be confined to certain predetermined areas of the planning region.

In addition to the constraints listed above, there can be some other constraints which might require upper bounds on the waiting times of certain facilities, upper bounds on the travel time for certain sections of the population, the exclusion of certain areas from consideration as possible sites for certain facilities, and the exclusion of certain design classes in some proposed facilities. It is also possible that a predetermined upper bound on the total cost will result in the elimination of some feasible solutions.

The planning model will minimize the total cost of primary health care by optimizing the arrangement of facility characteristics and locations.

Algorithm for Optimization

Because of a large number of decision variables, and the broad range of values for each variable, complete enumeration of all feasible solutions is virtually impossible. In this case, a number of optimization techniques [15] can be applied for obtaining an optimal solution. Some of these techniques are nonlinear programming, dynamic programming, and heuristic optimization. Even with simple attractiveness functions, the cost function is composed of a very large number of terms with polynomials in the numerator as well as denominator of each term. It is extremely difficult to ascertain whether this function is convex or concave, unimodal or nonunimodal. Therefore, the commonly used nonlinear programming techniques cannot be expected to work efficiently. Dynamic programming is ruled out because of a very large number of state variables.

A heuristic optimization technique does not guarantee an optimal solution, but it does provide an efficient approach to the evaluation of a number of feasible solutions. A properly selected heuristic algorithm can lead to a suboptimal solution, which can be a good approximation to the optimal solution. Since it is practically impossible to obtain an optimal solution, in the current situation a heuristic algorithm was developed.

The algorithm for optimizing the cost function in this model is based on the direct-search decision rule for converging on the optimum through a series of suboptimal solutions, in which the latest solution is better than the preceding solution. The algorithm starts with a trial solution in which the characteristics of all facilities are defined along with the coordinates of the proposed facilities. If the trial solution is not feasible, an attempt is made to generate a feasible solution. If no feasible solution can be obtained, the next trial solution is taken up. If a feasible solution is obtainable, an effort is made to get a better solution. This movement toward a better solution goes on until certain conditions for the termination of the algorithm exist, and the algorithm is terminated for the trial under consideration. In this manner, all the trials are gone through, and the best result is recorded.

In the "planning model," the coordinates of various population centers and facilities are restricted to integer values to speed up the process of optimization. If the size of a coordinate unit is sufficiently small (0.2 mile in 10,000 square miles of planning territory), this restriction will not introduce any significant error in the computation of total cost.

A small test problem is presented in Appendix 3A. A detailed flowchart and a tape of the computer routine for the model can be obtained from NTIS [1]. This model can handle problems involving a maximum of 99 population centers, 48 existing facilities, 20 proposed facilities, and 9999 coordinates along either axis of reference.

References

1. Harpal Dhillon and Richard J. Giglio, *A Computer Model for Planning Locations, Capacities and Schedules of Outpatient Facilities*, Report Number UMASS/IEOR-77/2 (Springfield, VA.: U.S. Department of Commerce, National Technical Information Service, 1977).

2. William J. Abernathy and John G. Hershey, "A Spatial-Allocation Model for Regional Health Service Planning," *Operations Research*, vol. 20, no. 3 (May-June 1972).

3. R.L. Bashshur, G.W. Shannon, and C.A. Metzner, "The Concept of Distance as a Factor in Accessibility and Utilization of Health Care," *Medical Care Review* 26:143-61, 1969.

4. L.J. Shuman, C.P. Hardwick, and G.A. Huber, "Location of Ambulatory Care Centers in a Metropolitan Area," *Health Services Research* 8(2):121-38, 1973.

5. A. Ciocco and I. Altman, "Medical Service Areas and Distances Travelled for Physician Care in Western Pennsylvania," U.S. Public Health Service, Public Health Monograph No. 19, 1959.

6. Harpal S. Dhillon, "A Quantitative Analysis of the Influence to Time Factors on the Spatial Distribution of Non-Emergency Health Care Facilities," Ph.D. dissertation, University of Massachusetts, 1974.

7. J.W. Lubin, D.L. Drosness, and L.G. Wylie, "Highway Network Minimum Path Selection Applied to Health Facility Planning," *Public Health Reports* 80:33, 1965.

8. W.J. Abernathy, J.R. Moore, and E.L. Schrens, "Distance and Health Services: Issues of Utilization and Facility Choice for Demographic Strata," Research Paper No. 19, Stanford University, Graduate School of Business, July 1971.

9. R.D. Coughlin, "Hospital Complex Analysis: An Approach to Analysis for Planning a Metropolitan System of Service Facilities," Ph.D. dissertation, University of Pennsylvania, 1964.

10. J. Schneider, "Measuring the Locational Efficiency of the Urban Hospital," *Health Services Research* 2:154, Summer 1967.

11. C.S. Revelle and R.W. Swain, "Central Facilities Location," *Geographic Analysis* 2:30, January 1970.

12. C. Toregas, C. Revelle, R. Swain, and L. Bergman, "The Location of Emergency Service Facilities," *Operations Research* 19:1363, October 1971.

13. Edward J. Rising, *Ambulatory Care Systems, Vol. I: Design for Improved Patient Flow* (Lexington, MA.: Lexington Books, 1977).

14. N.T.J. Bailey, "A Study of Queues and Appointment Systems in Hospital Outpatient Departments with Special Reference to Waiting Times," *Journal of Royal Statistical Society* (B), 14, 1952.

15. H.M. Wagner, *Principles of Operations Research*, 2d ed. (Englewood Cliffs, N.J.: Prentice-Hall, 1975).

Appendix 3A:
Sample Problem

In this test problem, the following information is assumed.

Number of existing population centers 4

Number of proposed population centers 1

Number of existing facilities 6

Number of proposed facilities 2

The coordinates of both the facilities are bounded. In the subsequent presentation, the following symbols will be used.

K	Index(code) number for a facility
NHX(K)	X coordinate of facility K
NHY(K)	Y coordinate of facility K
HTV(K)	Number of user-visits per period expected at facility K
NARANK(K)	Facility rank[a] for facility K

Initial Trial Solution

K	NHX(K)	NHY(K)	NARANK(K)
1	211	321	10
2	140	201	9
3	85	253	12
4	271	201	10
5	135	95	12
6	231	275	13
7[b]	85	320	7
8[b]	180	195	7

The initial solution was not feasible because facility number 6 was overloaded.

---

[a]In this model, NARANK(K) represents the rank of facility number. The rank number corresponds to a combination of facility operational characteristic and physical characteristics.
[b]Proposed facility.

First Feasible Solution

K	NHX(K)	NHY(K)	NARANK(K)	HTV(K)
1	211	321	10	1976
2	140	201	9	3712
3	85	253	12	3523
4	271	201	10	3339
5	135	95	12	4668
6	231	275	14	6659
7	85	320	7	2935
8	180	195	7	1986

Note: The feasible solution is obtained by changing the ranks of the proposed facilities. Facility coordinates cannot be changed.

Cost Estimates

The following cost estimates were obtained for the first feasible solution.

Service cost per period	$ 499,400.00
Inconvenience cost per period	$ 203,766.00
Total cost per period	$ 703,166.00

Iteration Toward the Best Solution for This Trial

The iteration process began with a step size of 20 coordinate units for each proposed facility. For this trial, the terminal step size was 1 coordinate unit, and the step size factor was set at 2.0.

Best Solution for This Trial

K	NHX(K)	NHY(K)	NARANK(K)	HTV(K)
1	211	321	10	1983
2	140	201	9	3162
3	85	253	12	2971
4	271	201	10	3358
5	135	95	12	3855
6	231	275	14	6673

K	NHX(K)	NHY(K)	NARANK(K)	HTV(K)
7	63	354	7	2745
8	158	194	7	4051

Cost Estimates

The following cost estimates were obtained for the best solution for this trial.

Service cost per period	$ 499,400.00
Inconvenience cost per period	$ 191,339.00
Total cost per period	$ 690,737.90

Attractiveness Functions

In the test problem, the following attractiveness function was used.

$$A_{i,j} = \frac{1}{a(t_{i,j})^b + c(W_j - \overline{W})^d}$$

where

$A_{i,j}$ = probability of a resident of population center i being attracted to facility j

$t_{i,j}$ = perceived travel time for traveling from population center i to facility j

w_j = average waiting time for a user of facility j

$\overline{W}$ = average waiting time for all facilities in the subregion. (The planning region was divided into three subregions, based on the population density; this was necessary because the conceptual measures of convenience seemed to be related to where the population center is located.)

a, b, c, d = parameters which were estimated on the basis of empirical data (There was one set of parameters for each subregion.)

Part II:
Planning the Layout
of an Ambulatory
Care Facility

Introduction

The purpose of Part II (Chapters 4 and 5) is to present some general guidelines on how to plan the layout of a facility for delivering outpatient care. These guidelines should be helpful to business managers, physicians, or other parties who have had little or no prior experience in planning layouts. Although the emphasis is placed on planning a layout for an outpatient facility which provides a comprehensive range of services (such as an HMO), these guidelines are equally suited for specialized clinics or those offering a limited number of services. Since this section is not intended to be a comprehensive technical design guide, it should be used in conjunction with the services of an architect and the desires of the local community and other parties with a stake in the facility.

The guidelines encompass only part of the planning process, and it is strongly suggested that they be used within the context of a master plan which states the overall goals of the facility and the ways in which these goals can be met. For example, a goal might be to operate a clinic which stresses family care, which is designed to serve a particular community, or which is intended to suit the interests of a group of physicians. Compromises in facility design often have to be made—the most acceptable compromises will be those made with the guidance of a master plan. A master plan will guide the choice of a site and state the overall design philosophy. Also, if it has been determined that phased building of the facility is desirable from a cost standpoint, it is advisable to have a master plan that includes the relationship and connection of the secondary phase to the first phase. A master plan is discussed more fully elsewhere [1].

Part II addresses two questions: How large should the service areas of a particular facility be? and How should they be arranged in relation to each other? It is assumed that the preliminary investigation and planning have already taken place. In particular, it is assumed that:

1. A design committee has been chosen and has been involved in the initial stages of planning. It is recommended that representatives of the facility staff become involved in the design process. Generally, a design committee is responsible for several different functions. For example, a design committee might include an architect, business manager, owners, representatives of the staff, and members of the community to be served.
2. An architect has been chosen. Generally, an architect's services would have been used during the preliminary investigations of the site and possibly during discussions concerning services to be provided and expected growth patterns. The architect will be responsible for converting the wishes of the design committee concerning functional relationships into a schematic

The author wishes to acknowledge the contributions of David Rumpf, Ph.D. to Chapters 4 and 5.

design that shows all the rooms, their suggested locations, and their dimensions. Furthermore, the architect will describe an appropriate esthetic environment.

3. A site has been chosen, or at least some candidate sites have been selected. The final design must take into account any restrictions imposed by a particular site, and thus decisions regarding location and facility design often must be made concurrently.

4. The services which will be provided and the expected patient volume and its pattern of growth have been determined.

The services to be provided and the expected patient demand form the basis for the design process. If more detailed information is desired on how to determine the services to be provided, the expected patient volume, and the expected pattern of growth, or if the facility is in the initial stages of planning, one can consult other guides [1, 2].

Chapter 4 presents *general guidelines* for determining the size of service areas and a *procedure* for determining their relative placement (layout). Chapter 5 lists *specific recommendations* for the placement of most service areas in a health facility for use as a check on the design decisions arrived at in Chapter 4, as well as for general guidance. These recommendations have been compiled from various design guides published in North America and the United Kingdom and from discussions with facility managers.

References

1. Richard Miller, et al., *The Health Maintenance Organization Facility Development Handbook* (Rockville, MD.: U.S. Department of Health, Education and Welfare, Bureau of Community Health Services, 1974).

2. John R. Coleman and Frank C. Kaminsky, *Ambulatory Care Systems, Volume IV: Designing Medical Services for Health Maintenance Organizations* (Lexington, MA.: Lexington Books, 1977).

4 Determining the Size and Placement of Service Areas

Steps in the Planning Process

The steps involved in the proposed method for planning the size and physical layout of clinic are listed below and discussed in detail on the following pages.

1. Determine goals and objectives.
2. Determine a target year.
3. Prepare a list of all expected activity sequences for the current and target years.
4. Prepare traffic flow diagrams for all expected activity sequences.
5. Determine the load on each service area.
6. Determine the number and size of rooms required for each service area.
7. Specify the relative placement of service areas (proximity chart).
8. Prepare a bubble design.
9. Prepare a schematic design.

One individual, usually a high-level administrator, should be responsible for planning, although many of the tasks can be delegated. The administrator will have to interact regularly with the design committee, of course.

Determine Goals and Objectives

Since a facility is constructed to meet certain goals and satisfy various objectives, these goals and objectives should be determined and ranked in order of priority before the actual design process is started. In this context, *goals* relate to the underlying philosophy of a facility, while *objectives* correspond to the more specific aims of facility operation. The goals and objectives will provide a guide for all stages of the design, construction, and operation of the facility. The goals and objectives of an organization may seem obvious and their enumeration a waste of time. However, different individuals inevitably assign differing priorities to objectives, and unless these differences are made explicit, it may be difficult to arrive at a consensus with regard to a plan.

A possible set of goals and objectives for a facility is presented below. The list is not meant to be exhaustive and should be expanded or contracted according to the philosophy and desires of a particular design committee.

Goals:
> To provide the best health care that resources will permit
> To serve a particular community

Objectives:
> Minimize patient waiting time
> Satisfy patient and staff preferences
> Minimize cost
> Minimize patient traffic and staff movement
> Satisfy constraints of site, existing building laws and state codes
> Eliminate unnecessary traffic through clinics
> Satisfy communication needs within the facility
> Provide patient education
> Act as a community center

The goals of a clinic often will be contradictory. For example, patient waiting time can often be reduced only by scheduling fewer patients or adding more staff, actions which increase costs. Therefore, goals should be assigned a priority. Managers can go even one step further if they wish to be more precise; they can quantify goals. For example, they might specify that average waiting time will not exceed 20 minutes with no more than 10 percent of the patients waiting more than 35 minutes. Unfortunately, the quantitative measurement of goals involves data collection by observation and questionnaires as well as validation studies. The state of the art of the management of health care facilities is not yet well developed and so such efforts are usually expensive.

We suggest that most clinics can make decisions with only the priority listing of goals, along with a description of how layout affects the achievement of each goal.

Then when compromises are necessary during the planning process, the goals and objectives should be used as guidelines for the final compromises agreed upon by the design committee. There are techniques [3] for helping resolve conflicts and for clarifying goals which planners might find useful in making compromises.

Determine a Target Year

The determination of the initial size of a planned facility is usually based on an analysis of the expected level of patient demand at a specified period in the future or, more precisely, during the *target year*. The choice of a target year on which to base the size of a facility is generally governed by economic factors. Planning a facility based on the expected demand and staffing for the first year of operation is usually shortsighted, unless most of the patient load is being transferred from an existing practice. On the other hand, a target year beyond the fifth year of operation could involve too many uncertainties to be useful in determining facility size.

Since each facility will have its own unique characteristics, there is no universal procedure for determining an optimal target year. Some of the factors which influence the choice of a target year are given below.

Reasons for choosing a late target year (build all capacity now)	*Reasons for choosing an early target year (frequent expansions)*
It is less expensive to add more space during initial construction.	There is no expense (interest on capital, maintenance, utilities) on space which is not yet needed.
Construction costs are increasing.	There is less risk of inaccurate forecasts resulting in an inappropriate facility.
Expansion disrupts the facility.	

It is possible to calculate [3, 4] the optimal target year and both the initial size and future expansions for a facility. Such a calculation requires forecasts of demand growth, interest rates, various costs, and the rate of inflation. Many mathematical models exist for making such a calculation and, depending on the quality of the forecasts and the perseverance of the analyst, the models can be extremely accurate. Appendix 4A presents a rudimentary model which is recommended for determining the optimal target year. If planners do not wish to use the technique we suggest, they should use a target year of 4 to 5 years.

Provided the option of expansion has not been precluded by site considerations or the design of the building, additions can be made at a later date if warranted. Since it is difficult to conduct long-term planning for a facility without considering external factors such as the construction of competing facilities, local population changes, etc., long-term planning should usually be done on a regional basis.

Prepare List of All Expected Activity Sequences for the Current and Target Years

An *activity sequence* can be defined as the set of actions and movements made by patients and/or staff members for specific types of functions performed in the facility. For example, an activity sequence involving a patient and staff members will arise when a patient reports for a particular type of visit (i.e., a dental health visit). Also, an activity sequence can occur when a staff member performs a certain function that does not directly involve a patient. The identification of all major expected activity sequences is required in order to conduct a traffic flow analysis for the facility (see next step). Examples of sequence types are shown in Table 4-1. The list of activity sequences should include all types expected—initially and for the "target" year.

Table 4-1
A Checklist of Examples of Activity Sequences

Health Care Services Visits (involving patients and staff)
    Appointment care
    Nonappointment care
    Off-hours care
    Ancillary services visit
    Group appointments (family, etc.)
    Physical therapy care
    Mental health care
    Dental care
    Vision care
    OB/Gyn care

Administrative Services Visits (patients and staff)
    Patient enrollment
    Information requests
    Patient complaints
    Patient appointments

Specific Patient Functions
    Prescription pickup
    Laboratory visit
    Radiology visit

Staff Functions (staff only)
    Medical education

Miscellaneous
    Accompanying children and adults
    Visitors
    Health education
    Community/Consumer meetings
    Sales representatives' visits
    Employment applicants
    Deliveries of supplies

Prepare Traffic Tables

One method of obtaining the most effective use of space relies on the preparation of tables which show the movements made by patients and staff for each major activity sequence. Table 4-2 contains an example of a worksheet completed for a patient who comes to the facility for a nonappointment visit. By completing this traffic flow analysis, one can develop the circulation pattern of a facility [5].

The worksheet of Table 4-2 contains a list of most of the service areas which will be included in a facility and shows their approximate usage for an example service visit. Although often it will be difficult to estimate an accurate percentage to place in the "Use" column of Table 4-2, the planner's best guess can still provide valuable information. Studies of existing facilities can be used to estimate percentages when the planner is unable to supply this information. It is most important that these tables be complete, and the cooperation of the staff is essential when the diagrams are being prepared.

A worksheet similar to that of Table 4-2 should be constructed for staff movements for major types of service visits. Physician movements are normally limited to only a subset of service areas (examination rooms, consultation rooms, medical records, etc.), so all the service areas of Table 4-2 are normally not required.

Determine the Load on Each Service Area

If the expected patient volume for the health facility has not yet been broken down by type of service visit, this should be accomplished now.

Since the worksheet in Table 4-2 will have been completed for all major types of service visits by planing percentages in the "Use" column, it is possible to estimate the number of people who will use each service area in a year, day, or other appropriate time interval. The procedure is simply to multiply the number of visits by the percentage of time the particular area is used. For example, if 40 visits in the category "nonappointment care" are expected each day, then the main entrance area will be used 80 percent $\times$ 40, or about 36 times per day, for that particular type of visit. By summarizing the types of service visits, the daily load on the main entrance is easily calculated. A table such as in Table 4-3 can help facilitate this computation. Similar tables should be constructed for physician and nurse traffic.

The planner must keep in mind that the accuracy of the percentages estimated in the traffic worksheet will limit the accuracy of the entire procedure. However, even if the method offers results which are only approximate, it will be a valuable aid for space planning.

Table 4-2
Patient Traffic Worksheet

Filled out for: Example Visit, Nonappointment Care Visit

Service Area/Place	Percentage Use	Remarks
Common		
Entrance	80%	Regular hours
Off-hours entrance	20%	Off hours
Main reception	75%	Regular hours
Main waiting		
Subwaiting (specify)	100%	Nonappointment care waiting area
Medical records	100%	Need access during off hours
Transcription		
Library		
Conference		
Lounge/dining		
Lockers/employee facilities		
Receiving		
Storage–central supply		
Security		
Appointments	35%	
Other services (health, education, nutrition, etc.–specify)	10%	
Maintenance		
Switchboard		
Discharge	100%	If facility has a separate discharge
Administration		
Administrator		
Subscriber office		
Enrollment office		
Business office		
Purchasing		
Comptroller/accounting		
Machine room		
Medical director		
Nursing director		
Personnel		
Marketing		
Insurance		
General medicine		
Internal medicine		
Pediatrics		

Table 4-2 (cont.)

Service Area/Place	Percentage Use	Remarks
Medicine		
OB/Gyn		
Consulting medical specialty (specify)	12%	
Consulting surgical specialty (specify)	6%	
Radiology	18%	
Laboratory	20%	
Optometry		
Pharmacy	40%	
Dentistry		
Family planning		
Mental health	7%	
Nurse practitioner	60%	Depending on operating policies of facility
Other (specify)		

Determine Number and Size of Rooms Required for Each Service Area

The process of deciding on the number and size of rooms for each service area is difficult. The design committee will necessarily be making compromises involving cost, philosophy of patient care, expansion requirements, privacy, patient waiting, staff preferences, utilization, and security of the facility. These compromises should be agreed upon openly and made in terms of the master plan for the facility.

At this stage, one should be sure that a copy of local building codes is available and that sections relevant to physical layout have been studied. Of special interest are the restrictions on room sizes, specifications on exits and stairways, and restrictions on the proximity of various areas to one another.

Table 4-3
Summary Sheet of Patient Traffic in Service Areas

Period (day, year, etc.)	Visits per Period, % Use (from Table 4-2) X Number of Visits					
Service Area/Place	Enrollment	Information	First Visit	Nonappointment	etc.	Total
Entrance						
Off-Hours Entrance						
etc.						
Total						

The process of determining the number and sizes of rooms and service areas consists of four steps.

1. Determine approximate room sizes.
2. Based on demand and staffing, determine the number of examination and consultation rooms for each medical service area.
3. Based on demand and staffing, determine the number and type of rooms for ancillary and support service areas. These areas include:
    Radiology
    Medical lab and EKG
    Support services
        Health education
        Nutrition
        Public health
        Social services
    Medical records
    Centralized appointment/communication services
    Public areas
    General clinic services
    Clinic administration
    Vision care
    Mental health
    Dental care
    Outpatient pharmacy
    Plan administration
4. Estimate the gross area from net area.

Each of the four steps is discussed in turn.

(1) *Determine the room sizes.* The optimal size of an examination room, consultation room, or waiting room, etc., is a function of many factors. These factors include staff preferences, building codes, patient comfort, cost, and, of course, the activities which go on inside the room. The design committee must consider the factors affecting each service area and include them in the design process. In general, the final design will involve several compromises and should have the approval of all concerned. To facilitate determination of room size, suggestions of room size for various specialty areas are provided in Table 4-4.

In general, a room should be as small as possible and still allow space for equipment and for the staff to perform their duties. Consequently, for each type of room, the following questions should be asked:

What equipment will be in the room?

What are the equipment dimensions?

What is the maximum number of staff who will be in the room at one time?

How many clients will be in the room at a single time?

What activities will take place in the room? That is:

> What pattern of movement is exhibited by both the doctor and the patient inside the room?

> Will the doctor use the examination room for consultation?

> Will the examination room be useful for different specialties?

> If so, what are these specialties?

> Are there any special characteristics of the patients or activities performed in the room?

Based on the above information and the use of templates or via a simulated examination, the design staff can determine the approximate minimal dimensions for a room.

The minimal dimensions can be expanded if the staff feels uncomfortable in rooms of that size—provided there are sufficient funds. Patient comfort and relaxation are also a prime consideration in the determination of room size. Fortunately, there is evidence to suggest that patients who spend only a relatively short time in an examination room prefer small rooms for the feeling of privacy that they offer. Consequently, except for a waiting room, patient preferences would not argue for rooms much larger than the minimum determined by function.

Shannon has recommended the use of a 9 X 13 ft module (and its multiples) as the basic room size for a medical facility [6]. He warns that the design committee as a whole must agree to the modular concept and the size of the module. The advantages of this approach are most apparent in future expansion when a department moves to a larger area and a new specialty moves into the original location.

(2) *Determine the number of examination and consultation rooms required.* An examination room is required for each doctor. A consultation room is also required, allowing the doctor to talk with a patient or with members of the patient's family about confidential matters. Privacy, relaxation, and comfort have to be considered in the interior design of the consultation room. Although in some instances an examination and consultation room can be the same room, this is not currently common practice.

Determining the optimal number of examination rooms for a facility can be a complex undertaking. This is because the optimal number will depend, among other things, upon the staffing, types of specialties, the variation in work load, the way staff members are scheduled, and the work habits of the physicians. However, there are some generally accepted rules of thumb which can be used as guidelines. These rules of thumb are not meant to be absolutes, and the planner should not hesitate to violate them provided he or she has a documented reason for doing so.

Table 4-4
Checklist of Room Sizes [1]

Room	Suggested Square Feet	Minimum Square Feet	Maximum Square Feet	Minimum Recommended Dimension, Feet
General Medicine, Pediatrics, OB/Gyn, Consulting Surgery, Dermatology, Neurology				
Exam[a]	100	55	150	7
Consult	120	80	175	8
Exam/Consult[a]	125	85	155	8
Nurse station	60	40	190	6
Utility	50	45	115	7
Treatment	120	90	185	9
Office	90	50	135	7
Workroom	90	55	120	6
Supply	20	10	90	5
Toilet[b]	20	20	25	4
Nonappointment				
On call	130	120	150	9
Radiology				
Office	100	80	130	8
Reception[c]		60	110	7
Darkroom	60	30	105	6
Workroom	90	60	120	8
Procedure		205	295	12
Dressing	20	10	30	3
Barium	75	50	100	5
Allergy				
Exam[a]	100	100	140	8
Consult	85	80	85	8
Utility	50	40	65	7
Injection	50	35	55	7
Opthalmology				
Exam[a]	100	80	230	10
Consult	90	85	90	8
Exam/Consult[a]	125	115	155	10
Orthopedics				
Exam/Consult[a]	130	125	170	8
Storage		30	115	4

Table 4-4 (cont.)

Room	Suggested Square Feet	Minimum Square Feet	Maximum Square Feet	Minimum Recommended Dimension, Feet
Laboratory				
Exam	90	30	150	7
Office	90	55	165	7
Laboratory	200	100	820	11
Supply	40	30	45	6
Specimen collection	60	25	130	5
Dental				
Exam/Treat[a]	110	55	165	8
Darkroom	70	30	110	5
Workroom	80	20	105	8
Laboratory	60	60	60	6
Pharmacy				
Office	60	55	65	7
Dispensing				
Clinic with 40,000 visits/year	200			
Clinic with 80,000 visits/year	500			
Clinic with 120,000 visits/year	700			
Storage				
Clinic with 40,000 visits/year	100			
Clinic with 80,000 visits/year	200			
Clinic with 120,000 visits/year	300			
Psychiatry				
Consult	120	85	150	9
Office	120	100	135	8
Observation	200	100	250	10
Administration				
Office	150	100	200	10
Clerk space	60	50	100	
Common				
Entrance	100			
Reception	80/ receptionist			10

Table 4-4 (cont.)

Room	Suggested Square Feet	Minimum Square Feet	Maximum Square Feet	Minimum Recommended Dimension, Feet
Waiting area: should hold 85% of the capacity for a session	15/20 seat			
Circulation	300			
Supply: scattered throughout the service areas		20	500	4
Appointment	100+50/clerk			
Switchboard	100/operator			
Toilets:				
mens'	90			
womens'	90			
Physical Therapy				
Consult	100	50	120	8
Treatment	100	100	300	7
Exercise		150	330	15
Hydrotherapy		70	160	8
Screening				
Office	60	55	65	7
Exam[a]		75	125	7
ENT				
Exam	100	80	115	7
Audio	40	30	40	5
Medical Records				
Record Space	50/10,000 records			
Clerical	60/file clerk			
Supply	100			
Physicians' lounge	100 ft² + 20 ft²/physician on duty at one time			
Central sterilization	120			6
Maintenance services		40	200	6
General stores		40	200	6
Housekeeping services	40/8 physicians			
Service entrance	100	80	200	8

Table 4-4 (cont.)

Room	Suggested Square Feet	Minimum Square Feet	Maximum Square Feet	Minimum Recommended Dimension, Feet
Heating, ventilation, air conditioning, services		500	1300	
Other Areas				
Garage				
Elevators				
Stairways				

[a]Local code may control area or dimension.
[b]Toilet facilities should be convenient to all service areas.
[c]See section on "Common" areas.

Although a clinic may be open 16 or 24 hours per day, there is one period of maximum usage which determines the size and number of rooms that should be used. Normally, this period is during the working day when the maximum number of patients is scheduled and the maximum number of staff is present. A general rule of thumb for primary-care physicians is the use of two examination rooms for each physician on duty at the time of peak load. In this way, a physician can be examining a patient in one room while another patient is being readied in another. Times will arise when the physician could utilize more than two; for example, one room could be taken by a patient who is being treated by a nurse, the second by the physician himself, and the third by a patient getting ready. But in general, except for pediatrics where three rooms are recommended, two examination rooms per physician should suffice for the peak load period.

There are some specialties which require very little room preparation and clean up (for example, counseling in mental health), and therefore an average of less than two examination rooms per professional should suffice. However, there should always be more examination rooms than clinical professionals so that the likelihood of having a clinician and a patient waiting for an empty examination room is slight. Since the yearly operating and amortization cost of even a fully equipped examination room is small compared to staff salaries, there are also economic considerations involved in using extra examination rooms.

For example, a 10 × 10 ft examination room costing an incremental amount of $80/ft^2 to build and furnished with $10,000 worth of equipment results in a capital cost of $18,000. Amortizing that over the life of the building and including incremental costs for heat, maintenance, etc., would still result in a cost of no more than $2500 per year for that particular room. Since the cost of the physician for a year may be 20 times that, it is clear that the tradeoff between more rooms and physician waiting-time costs is heavily in favor of more rooms.

A planner may be particularly concerned with space utilization because of extenuating circumstances such as being forced to make use of inappropriate or cramped quarters. In this case, the problem of determining the number of examination rooms can be studied using cost-benefit techniques of the type briefly mentioned above. However, such a straightforward analysis may not be realistic because room usage varies by time of day, medical specialty, and patient. Consequently, it may be necessary to use techniques which take into account the probabilities of certain happenings, such as the simulation used in Reference 7 which takes into account the complicated usage patterns which can arise.

Another way to look into the question of how many examination rooms are required is to analyze data from existing practices which give the ratios of examination to consultation rooms. Table 4-5 lists the high, low, and median number of examination rooms per consultation room for five specialty areas. This information was collected from twelve different outpatient medical facilities [1].

Another recommendation to consider at this stage is the combination of two or more specialty areas into one design unit by the use of common examination and consultation rooms. This is particularly useful for specialty areas which have a low expected patient volume or which can be set up on alternative day or morning versus afternoon schedules. It may provide less privacy for the individual physician, but the benefits in relation to the cost can be substantial. Also, it is possible to build in flexibility by having one or more examination rooms between two specialty areas so the rooms can serve a dual purpose [8]. One noteworthy design of an examination room is the Mayo clinic's examination room [9] where the doctor's office is included in the examination room.

In an interesting variation of the Mayo model, all examination rooms have enough furniture to make adequate, if spartan, consultation rooms. In addition, pairs of physicians share an office which is not used for consultation with patients. Such an arrangement provides space for books and belongings while fostering interchange and collegiality among staff members. In at least one setting physicians preferred this arrangement to the more traditional approach.

Table 4-5
Number of Examination Rooms per Consultation Room

Specialty	High	Low	Median
Medicine or general practice	3.4	1.1	2.0
Pediatrics	3.8	1.5	2.3
OB/Gyn	2.0	1.0	1.6
Consulting surgical specialist	4.0	2.0	2.1
Consulting medical specialist	4.0	1.5	1.8

If two or more physicians share a number of examination rooms, a system of different colored lights over doorways can be used to indicate where a patient is waiting for a particular doctor. If indicators are wired to the physician's office, they can serve as a call system. Also, the state of the lights can be displayed at the switchboard, thereby making it possible to locate a physician easily in the event of an emergency.

(3) *Determine the number of rooms for ancillary and support service areas.* Although most physicians work best with two examination rooms, two rooms are not needed for all specialties. Each specialty should propose a basic design unit, showing the number and general relationship of their examination/ consultation rooms, laboratory facilities, toilets, conference rooms, waiting areas, etc. This design unit should not include any general or shared areas. Also, care should be taken to keep space requirements to a minimum. Some suggested guidelines are given below:

Radiology: When more than one technician is to be on duty at the same time, each should have his or her own examination/consultation room, control booth, dressing booth, and toilet. Each radiologist should have his own office. Other space can be shared by radiologists and technicians.

Medical Laboratory and EKG: Rapid advances in technology and the numerous services that can be provided make it difficult to estimate space requirements for medical laboratories. However, certain guidelines have been developed [10]. The U.S. Office of Economic Opportunity [11] suggests that a minimum of 400 ft^2 of laboratory space be provided for all new neighborhood health centers. This space would be used to provide a general laboratory for bacteriology, hematology, urinalysis, a venipuncture room, and a specimen room. In addition, another 50 ft^2 would be required for basal metabolism tests and electrocardiogram service.

Physical Therapy: Each therapist should have his or her own office. Also, treatment cubicles are required, and usually two will suit the needs of a clinic. In addition, an exercise area and an area with a whirlpool bath usually should be provided.

Mental Health: There should be an office for each of the peak number of psychiatrists, psychologists, social workers, and other therapists who will be on duty at one time. Area lavatories and a conference room are also required. Some facilities include an observation room. Depending on the type of treatment provided, the observation room and/or the conference room might be made large enough to hold group therapy sessions.

Dental: The dental suite should be designed so that there is at least one examination/treatment room for each hygienist who will be on duty at a given time. In addition, up to two treatment rooms for each dentist on duty at a given time should be available.

Vision Care: Each ophthamologist should have a separate consultation room and an examination/consultation room. Each optometrist needs one examination room.

(4) *Estimate the gross floor area*. Not all space in a building is usable for rooms and service areas. A sizable portion of the space is consumed by corridors, stairwells, mechanical shafts, ducts, elevators, and interior and exterior partitions. It has been estimated by architects that from 35 to 70 percent of the total area of medical buildings is unusable [1, 12]. The percentage of unusable area varies by organizational component and also by building type.

The concept of usable versus unusable area in health facilities has been expressed in terms of the ratio of net to gross area. *Gross area* can be defined as the total building area while *net area* refers only to room and service area space and excludes corridors, stairwells, etc. To avoid possible confusion in the use of these terms, the planner should realize that they are not universally used and that other people may employ a different basis for making this type of measurement.

Table 4-6 contains a breakdown of the percent of net to gross areas by organizational component for a sample of twelve facilities. Along organizational lines, the median percent of net area to gross area ranges from 67 percent for dental services to 91 percent for the lobby and pharmacy areas.

Table 4-6
Net-to-Gross Area for Various Organizational Components of Twelve HMOs [1]

Organizational Component	Low	High	Median
General Practice	63.3	76.3	69.4
Medical Specialties	69.4	85.5	78.7
Surgical Specialties	66.2	74.1	71.4
Pediatrics	67.6	75.2	72.0
Obstetrics	63.7	78.1	68.5
Psychiatry	68.5	90.9	76.9
Radiology	63.7	82.6	69.0
Laboratory	71.9	97.1	87.0
Pharmacy	84.7	97.1	90.9
Urgent Visit	65.8	81.3	71.9
Dental	62.5	78.1	67.1
Lobby	63.3	99.0	90.0
Supply	83.3	90.9	85.5
Administration	75.2	95.2	83.3

The planner should impress on the architect that, in addition to having the optimal sizes and number of rooms and service areas, the facility must have a high percentage of net to gross area. And 75 percent is not an unrealistic figure.

Specify the Relative Placement of All Service Areas

After completing steps 1 through 6, the design committee will have determined all expected service visits, which service areas they will utilize, what the expected volume of visits will be for each service area, and the size of each service area. This information can be used to construct a proximity chart (Figure 4-1) which indicates how close various service areas should be to one another.

To construct a proximity chart, the design committee should make the following lists.

	1	2	3	4	5	6	7	8	9	10
1 Waiting	1									
2 Reception	3	2								
3 Lab	2	1	3							
4 X-Ray	1	1	1	4						
5 Service Entrance	-1	-1	2	1	5					
6 Medical Records	2	3	2	1	0	6				
7 General Medical Exam	3	2	1	2	1	2	7			
8 Pharmacy	2	2	1	0	2	2	0	8		
9 Physical Therapy	2	2	0	0	1	2	1	0	9	
10										10

Closeness Rating	3	Proximity very desirable
	2	Proximity desirable
	1	Proximity preferable
	0	Proximity not important
	-1	Proximity undesirable

Figure 4-1. Example of a Proximity Chart.

Which service areas should be close to the main entrance? That is, which service areas:

(*a*) Have a high volume of expected service visits?

(*b*) Should be near the entrance for security and control (for example, the main reception point)?

Which service areas should be placed farther away from the main entrance? That is, which service areas:

(*a*) Have a relatively low volume of expected service visits?

(*b*) Are for staff use only, where privacy is desired?

(*c*) Would have a deleterious effect on the appearance of the clinic (for example, a loading ramp or storage area)?

Which service areas should be close to one another? That is, which service areas:

(*a*) Have high traffic flows between them—either patients or staff?

(*b*) Have a high potential for sharing examination rooms, equipment, etc.?

(*c*) Share common records?

(*d*) Have other reasons, based on the goals and objectives for a particular facility, for being close to one another?

Which service areas can be or should be separated from one another? That is, which service areas:

(*a*) Have a low volume of traffic flow between them?

(*b*) Need to be separated because of noise, contamination, staff privacy, security, etc.?

What service areas might be involved in future expansion and thus should be placed near an outer wall or designed for easy conversion to a new use?

As shown in Figure 4-1, the preparation of a proximity chart consists of listing all planned service areas along the left-hand side, drawing a triangle of boxes, and then using the information from the traffic flow diagrams and the above lists. Each box is filled in with the relationship that exists for the corresponding service areas. It may be desirable to redefine or expand on the "closeness" rating scale and include symbols on the chart giving the reasons behind the individual ratings.

Prepare Bubble Design

A bubble design shows the departmental and functional relationships in diagramatic form. It can also indicate site restrictions and expansion requirements. The usual approach is to have the bubble design prepared by an architect working from the information contained in the proximity chart. The result can then be discussed by the design committee with the architect and rearranged if desired. An example of a bubble design has been included for reference in Figure 4-2.

The design committee might find it helpful to prepare a bubble design independent of the architect's approach. This would help summarize the work that the design committee had accomplished up to this point as well as provide an excellent way to observe and openly decide upon any compromises which have to be made. One possible approach involves using a chalkboard, outlining

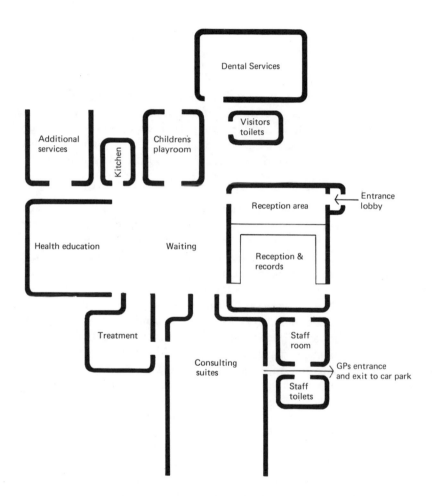

Adapted from: *Design Guide: Health Centers in Scotland*, Scottish Home and Health Development, Edinburgh, Scotland.

Figure 4-2. Example of Bubble Design Showing Room Relationships.

the site dimensions, and placing service areas into the site area using the proximity chart. One might prefer to use pieces of paper or plastic to represent each service area and attempt to find a good arrangement of the areas within an outline of the site (again using the lists and proximity chart). A more formal methodology is described in Appendix 4B.

Corridor placement should be indicated on the bubble design. Although corridor space should be kept to a minimum, adequate circulation space must be provided so the staff can visit all medical areas without passing through patient waiting areas.

Prepare Schematic Design

The schematic design will show all rooms, their proposed locations, and dimensions, and describe an appropriate physical environment. This design is obviously quite technical and should be prepared by an architect. A good working relationship with an architect is important since there will inevitably be decisions concerning the schematic design which will require consultation with other members of the design committee. A partial list of questions which may arise in this step follows.

1. How can one ensure the supervision of patients and security of the facility? This question is especially relevant for off-hours operations when there is a need for access to records and supplies as well as a requirement for security.
2. Should the facility have one main waiting area or several smaller waiting areas? Some obvious factors that affect this choice are the size of the facility, the diversity of service areas provided, and the objectives of the design committee, especially as regards the comfort of the waiting area, individualized attention, and costs. Some planners [6, 4] emphasize a maximum allowable distance of 30 yd from the reception point to the farthest examination room. Another guide [8] emphasizes the advantage of having one large but very pleasantly decorated waiting room, while another [1] emphasizes the importance of small, personally oriented waiting areas. In general, one large waiting room will utilize less space than several smaller rooms for a given number of people. However, a centralized room can take on the impersonal appearance of a bus terminal.
3. Who will prepare the signs to aid patient flow, and when will they be completed? Although it may seem to be a bit premature, the lack of signs can cause severe problems when a facility is opened and thus should be considered during the construction stage.
4. How much parking space should be provided? Here, the legal code requirements may determine the answer. A suggested rule of thumb is six parking places per physician [6].

5. If possible, should you buy more land adjacent to your present site? It should be remembered that the value of land near a successful clinic can become very expensive. It has been suggested [6] that 3 to 3 1/2 acres should be obtained for a facility initially housing 20 doctors.

References

1. Richard Miller, et al., *The Health Maintenance Organization Facility Development Handbook* (Rockville, MD.: U.S. Department of Health, Education and Welfare, Bureau of Community Health Services, 1974).

2. John R. Coleman and Frank C. Kaminsky, *Ambulatory Care Systems, Volume IV: Designing Medical Services for Health Maintenance Organizations* (Lexington, MA.: Lexington Books, 1977).

John R. Coleman and Frank C. Kaminsky, *Ambulatory Care Systems, Volume V: Financial Design and Administration of Health Maintenance Organizations* (Lexington, MA.: Lexington Books, 1977).

3. Edward J. Rising, Robert Baron, and Barry Averill, "A Systems Analysis of a University Health Service Outpatient Clinic," *Operations Research* 21, 5 (1973):1030.

4. Richard J. Giglio, "A Note on the Deterministic Capacity Problem," *Management Science* 19 (9):1096-99, 1973.

5. A.T. Kohler, Presentation at Group Health Institute, sponsored by the Group Health Foundation and Group Health Association of America, June 10, 1974.

6. William R. Shannon, "Architecture for Group Practice: Master Plan by Design," *Group Practice*, November 1970, 20-23.

7. Edward J. Rising, *Ambulatory Care Systems, Volume I: Design for Improved Patient Flow* (Lexington, MA.: Lexington Books, 1977).

8. G. Nedeljkob, *From the Family Doctor to the Medical Center: Problems of Organization* (Munich, Germany: Bauen and Wohnen, 1969).

9. R.W. Fleming, "Design of Outpatient Areas," *Hospital Topics*, October 1973.

10. U.S. Department of Health, Education, and Welfare, *Planning the Laboratory for the General Hospital*, Public Health Service Publication No. 930-D-10, U.S. Government Printing Office, Washington, D.C., November 1972.

11. *Space Guidelines for Ambulatory Health Centers*, Office of Health Affairs and the Facility Management Branch Procurement Division, OEO, Washington, D.C., November 1972.

12. *Design Guide: Health Centers in Scotland*, Scottish Home and Health Development, Her Majesty's Stationery Office, London, England.

Appendix 4A: Determining the Target Year

A determination of the target year requires data on construction costs, the expected inflation rate of construction costs, interest costs, and the growth rate of demand. Interestingly, although maintenance costs and the property tax rate will obviously affect the profitability of a facility, those quantities do not significantly affect the optimal target year. Methods for obtaining usable estimates of these are described below along with a formula for determining target years and sizes of capacity expansions. Some ability in mathematics is required to use the methodology.

Construction Costs

The architect or an engineering firm can supply estimates for various sizes of facilities. Estimates should be obtained for the smallest feasible size, the maximum size, and a size approximately midway in between. "Size" should be in the units of maximum visits per year which each facility can handle, and the estimates can be graphed as shown in Figure 4A-1.

Generally, the three estimates will not form a straight line because a larger facility does not cost proportionately more than a smaller one because of economies of scale. In order to use construction costs in the formula, they must be expressed in the form

$$\text{Cost } C = cx^{\alpha}$$

The parameters c and α are calculated by plotting costs on log-log graph paper, connecting the three points by the straight line which fits them best, and calculating c as the value where the line intercepts the C axis and α as the slope of the line. See Figure 4A-2.

Inflation Rate of Construction-Related Costs

The architect can supply an average for the expected inflation rate over the next 3 to 5 years. This rate also can be obtained from the *Engineering News Record.* Call the average yearly rate y.

Interest Rate

The interest rate for construction loans can be obtained from a bank. Denote this rate by i.

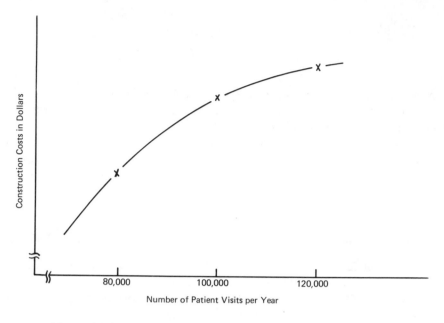

Figure 4A-1. Construction Costs as a Function of Patient-Visits.

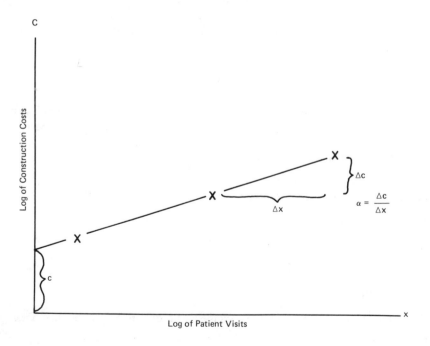

Figure 4A-2. Sample Construction Costs Plotted on Log-Log Paper.

Projected Demand

Estimated demand in terms of visits per year should be plotted for 5 or 10 years. Typically, demand projections will appear as shown in Figure 4A-3. The graph in Figure 4A-3, for example, reflects a situation where on opening day clients would arrive at the rate of 20,000 per year, after the first year they will be arriving at the rate of 40,000 visits per year, 55,000 per year after 3 years, and where demand will level off at about 60,000 visits per year after approximately 4 years. A curve of that form can be expressed by the mathematical function

$$D = d_0 + d(1 - e^{-gt})$$

where

D = demand in terms of visits per year
d_0 = demand now

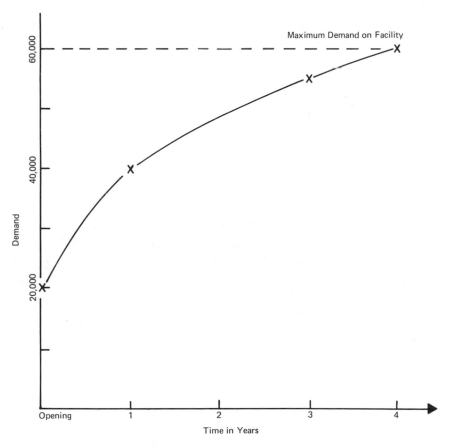

Figure 4A-3. Demand Projections.

t = time measured in years

d = maximum amount demand will grow above the level on opening day

g = parameter chosen to fit a particular growth pattern

For rapidly growing demand, g is relatively large; for slowly growing demand, g is relatively small. The values d_0, and d are available directly from the graph. There are numerous ways to calculate a value for g. Here we will suggest a simple trial-and-error procedure. Beginning with a value of $g = 0.5$, the function $D = d_0 + d(1 - e^{-gt})$ should be graphed as in Figure 4A-3. If it rises more quickly than the projected demand, a smaller value of g should be used on the next try; if it rises more slowly, a larger value should be used. After a few tries, a value of g will be found which gives a graph closely approximating expected demand.

Calculation Procedure

At this stage the planner will have calculated

Symbol	Explanation	Units or Comment
c	Construction cost factor	$/1000 visits/year
α	Construction cost factor	$0 < \alpha < 1$
y	Inflation rate	$\dfrac{\text{percent/year}}{100}$
i	Interest rate	$\dfrac{\text{percent/year}}{100}$
d_0	Current demand	visits/year
d	Maximum amount of demand above current level (maximum demand $= d_0 + d$)	visits/year
g	Demand-growth parameter	

Step 1. Calculate Effective Net Interest Rate r

$$r = i - y$$

If $r < 0$, the optimal policy is to build a facility now large enough to handle total demand of $d_0 + d$ visits per year.

Step 2. Calculate $B = r/g + \alpha$

If $B \leqslant 1$, then build $d_0 + d$ units of capacity now. That is, build the capacity sufficient to meet all anticipated demand. In other words, the target year is the far distant future.

If $B > 1$, build capacity at equally spaced intervals. The first capacity movement should be of size $X^* + d_0$ where X^* is such that

$$\alpha - \alpha \left(1 - \frac{X^*}{d}\right)^B - \frac{X^*}{d}B\left(1 - \frac{X^*}{d}\right)^{B-1} = 0$$

The target year is simply that year when demand is predicted to again equal existing capacity.

Finding the X^* satisfying the above equation is a trial-and-error process, and a simple computer routine could be programmed if the skills are available. Alternatively, a hand calculator could be used. Each successive capacity expansion should be $(1 - X^*/d)$ times the previous expansion.

Appendix 4B: Methodology for Determining Best Relationship between Service Areas

This appendix presents a method for obtaining a good "bubble design" or schematic placement of service areas in a facility by using the information summarized in the proximity chart. The schematic developed by facility planners can be then used by architects to develop detailed plans.

The analyst should prepare scale templates for each service area. A scale of ¼ in. to 1 ft is usually convenient. If the facility is to be installed in an existing building, a drawing to the same scale should be prepared for that building showing all fixed characteristics such as elevators, stairwells, windows, and entrances. These drawing and templates are then used in the procedure described below.

The procedure consists of two parts:

1. Using the proximity chart, an ordered list of the service areas is obtained. Areas highest on the list are the most critical in terms of placement.
2. The areas are then located relative to one another using the ordered list and the templates.

The procedure will be illustrated with the simple example whose proximity chart is given in Table 4B-1.

Table 4B-1
Proximity Chart of Example Problem

	W	R	L	X	S
Waiting (W)					
Reception (R)	3				
Lab (L)	2	1			
X-Ray (X)	1	1	1		
Service entrance/storage (S)	−1	−1	2	1	

Part 1: Obtaining an Ordered List of Areas

Step 1

Complete the proximity chart so it is a square rather than a triangle. This is done by noting that the chart is symmetrical so, for example, desirability of the

79

reception area being adjacent to the waiting area is the same as the desirability of adjacency of the waiting area and the reception room. For example, the proximity chart becomes

	W	R	L	X	S
W	–	3	2	1	−1
R	3	–	1	1	−1
L	2	1	–	1	2
X	1	1	1	–	1
S	−1	−1	2	1	–

Step 2

Sum up each column, *ignoring negative entries.* For example,

W	R	L	X	S
6	5	6	4	3

Step 3

Pick the column which has the largest sum. If more than one column has a sum equal to this number, just pick one of them arbitrarily. If no column has a sum greater than zero, go to step 8; otherwise continue. For example, columns W and L are tied with a sum of 6. Column W will be arbitrarily used.

Step 4

Examine that column for the largest element; if there exists several elements of the same size, arbitrarily pick one. For example, the largest element in column W is a 3 in row R. This particular 3 represents the desirability of having the reception area close to the waiting area.

Step 5

Place the selected proximity variable on a consecutive list. For example,

List
$$\overline{WR = 3}$$

Step 6

Replace the element just chosen and its mirror image with 0s on the proximity chart:

	W	R	L	X	S
W	—	0	2	1	−1
R	0	—	1	1	−1
L	2	1	—	1	2
X	1	1	1	—	1
S	−1	−1	2	1	—

Step 7

If the proximity chart is all 0s or (−1)s, go to step 8; otherwise go to step 2. One continues to go from steps 2 through 6 until the matrix has no positive entries and the list contains all service area combinations.

Step 2. Calculate column sums, ignoring negative entries.

W	R	L	X	S
3	2	6	4	3

Step 3. Choose the column with largest sum: column L sums to 6.

Step 4. Choose the largest element in the column chosen: Row W and row S equal 2; arbitrarily choose W.

Step 5. Add new combination to priority list:

List
WR = 3
WL = 2

Step 6. Replace the element chosen and its mirror image with 0s on the proximity chart:

	W	R	L	X	S
W	—	0	0	1	−1
R	0	—	1	1	−1
L	0	1	—	1	2
X	1	1	1	—	1
S	−1	−1	2	1	—

Step 7. If the matrix is all 0s or (−1)s, go to step 8; otherwise go to step 2.

Step 2. Calculate the column sums, ignoring negative entries.

W	R	L	X	S
1	2	4	4	3

Step 3. Choose the column with the largest sum: Columns L and X sum to 4; arbitrarily choose column L.

Step 4. Choose the largest element in the column chosen: Row S holds the largest element in column L.

Step 5. Add the new combination to the priority list:

List
WR = 3
WL = 2
LS = 2

Step 6. Replace the element chosen and its mirror image with 0s on the proximity chart:

	W	R	L	X	S
W	−	0	0	1	−1
R	0	−	1	1	−1
L	0	1	−	1	0
X	1	1	1	−	1
S	−1	−1	0	1	−

Step 7. If the matrix is all 0s or (−1)s, go to step 8; otherwise go to step 2. By continued iterations the following priority list would be generated (the calculations are omitted for reasons of space, but they take only a few moments).

List
WR = 3
WL = 2
LS = 2
WX = 1
RX = 1
LR = 1
XL = 1
XS = 1

At this point the table would be reduced to 0s or (−1)s, so one would go to step 8.

Step 8

End of part 1. Begin part 2.

Part 2: Solution Procedure

Step 9

Take the first set of service areas off the priority list. Using the templates, obtain a number of beginning layouts.

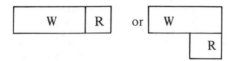

Step 10

Take each successive set of areas off the list. If a set has one or more areas in common with sets already taken off, it must be placed adjacent to the existing layout; otherwise it can be free-floating. Always make sure that area pairs with (−1)s are not adjacent. For example, add on WL:

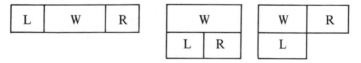

Add on LS:

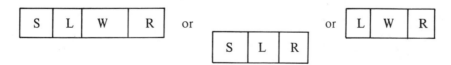

Add on WX:

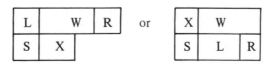

Add on RX:

X	W	
S	L	R

(difficulty in placing reception and X-ray adjacent)

Add on LR: already in place. Add on XL: already in place. Add on XS: already in place. One final solution:

X	W	
S	L	R

In the example, the procedure enabled one to obtain a bubble design which satisfies almost all the priorities placed on the relative locational service areas. For larger problems, the procedure is even more useful because it is difficult to visualize the best layout without some way to assign priorities to the placement of service areas.

5 Recommendations for the Placement of Service Areas in a Health Facility

This chapter contains some specific recommendations for the placement of various categories of service areas in a facility. These guidelines can serve as a check on layout decisions arrived at using the methods of Chapter 4 or when analytic techniques do not provide a clear indication for the placement of an area. The material has been compiled both from the literature and from private communications. For additional information concerning the factors involved in service area placement, one can consult Reference 1.

The suggestions of this chapter should be used with caution and interpreted in light of the goals and objectives of a particular facility. For example, a common rule of thumb specifies that as much as 2/3 to 1 ft^2 of overall building space will be needed per annual outpatient visit. Also, a widely used rule of thumb for outpatient facilities is the provision of 1000 to 1200 ft^2 of space per doctor. The planner should recognize that these figures are based on past experience and on existing designs and that they may not be useful in the development of a more efficient design.

In the following paragraphs each of the fifteen clinic functions has been classified into five main categories: reception and waiting, administration, patient treatment, other patient services, and service functions. The functions are listed below:

Reception and Waiting
1. Public Areas

Appointments and Records
2. Centralized appointment and communication system
3. Medical records

Patient Treatment
4. Physician services—family care area
5. Ancillary services—radiology, lab, physical therapy, EKG
6. Vision care
7. Mental health
8. Dental care
9. Surgery unit
10. Nonappointment care/urgent care clinic

Other Patient Services
11. Other medical support services—community area, public health, social worker, etc.
12. Outpatient pharmacy

Administration
13. Clinic administration
14. Plan administration

Service Functions
15. General clinic services

The reader will note that the fifteen functions listed above do not correspond exactly with the service areas listed in earlier sections of this book (e.g., Table 4-2). Rather, they are more general, and each can include a number of service areas. For the purpose of checking the general suitability of a design, a smaller number of service areas are easier to work with than a larger number. The design committee must, however, ensure that the layout of each service area is sound in addition to being concerned about the relationships among areas.

Table 5-1 lists a summary of recommendations. The suggested placement for each of the functions is given along with a brief rationale. Since the suggested placement for a majority of the service areas is near the general waiting area, we have devised a rating system. For example, the areas for clinic and plan administration and for centralized appointments should be close to the general waiting area. Since the administration area has a "2" priority, the centralized appointment area (which has a "1" priority) should be placed closer to the waiting area in the event of a conflict over space.

Public Areas

These include general waiting area, public toilets, and the reception point.

Suggested Placement: There are two conflicting positions taken on the placement of the waiting areas. The reception point should always be in a prominent position near the entrance. Some planners recommend a single general waiting area which includes the main entrance and reception point with nearby public toilets. An alternative plan, more suited to larger clinics, would be to have a general reception point with decentralized waiting areas for each clinic.

Rationale and Discussion: For the first alternative, the waiting room should be located so that all parts of it can be seen from the reception point. The reception point will receive patients, collect pertinent information, and arrange for orderly progress through the clinic. Since most patient treatment areas are located near the general waiting area, the traffic will be minimized, and very few separate

Table 5-1
Summary of Recommendations

Function	Suggested Placement	Rationale (Summarized)	Priorities[a]
Reception point, waiting, etc.	Prominent position near entrance	First point of patient contact with clinic	—
Centralized appointment area	Adjacent to general waiting area	Reappointments	1
Medical records	Convenient to appointment area and non-appointment care area	To facilitate access	3
Family care area	Adjacent to general waiting area	Minimize traffic	2
Ancillary service	Dependent on the type of service	Maximize ease of use by patients	2
Vision	Near general waiting area with separate access	Ease of patient movement	3
Mental health	Near general waiting area with separate access	Ease of patient movement	3
Dental care	Near general waiting and family care areas	Ease of patient movement	3
Surgery unit	Near radiology and non-appointment care	Proximity desired for medical reasons	3
Nonappointment care	Near main entrance	Comfort of other patients and security	3
Other medical	Near general waiting area with separate access	Separate access desirable	3
Outpatient pharmacy	Adjacent to main reception point	Facilitate prescription service	1
Clinic and plan	Near general waiting and reception area	Facilitate business appointments and plan interview	2
Clinic administration	Near general waiting and reception area	Facilitate business appointments and plan interview	2
General clinic services	Near separate entrance		

[a]Priority with respect to closeness to reception. Priority 1 is the highest.

waiting areas will be required. The patients will be called from the general waiting area into the appropriate clinic section. It is important that people are prevented from entering the medical area until the doctor or nurse is ready.

In the second alternative, the decentralized plan helps ensure that the distance between the waiting room and the farthest consultation room does not exceed 20 ft. The consultation and examination rooms should be arranged so that the distance between their waiting areas and the reception areas does not exceed 75 ft. (Other writers suggest that the longest walking distance from waiting area to examination room should be 90 ft [1].) Large central waiting rooms may be inconsistent with the concept of personalized care. In a health maintenance organization, waiting rooms designed to seat more than about 25 persons generally should require special justification [2]. Although it is desirable in many respects to have a central reception point at the entrance with separate clinic waiting areas, this arrangement does lead to queuing and delay at the main entrance and complicates the appointment system.

Some Other Considerations: A separate children's waiting area is sometimes beneficial. It has been found helpful to have a receptionist who can spend some time caring for children while their parents are in the examination room. When an outpatient clinic expects to have a large volume of severely handicapped patients (wheelchair or stretcher), it is advisable to provide an entrance separate from the heavy traffic of the main entrance.

The emphasis on multiclinic use of the general waiting area should encourage considerable attention to making this area a comfortable place both physically and psychologically. A pleasant environment can relieve boredom and anxiety. For example, comfortable seating can be arranged in a small conversational grouping. Furthermore, furniture should be easy to get into and out of (e.g., chairs and sofas which have arms).

Centralized Appointment and Communication Area

Suggested Placement: Adjacent to the general waiting area.

Rationale and Discussion: Patients may need to make reappointments at the time of their visit, and the appointment desk should be close to the waiting area to facilitate this process. The appointment area does not have to be the first contact point unless it is integrated with the reception, as it often is in a small facility.

Several studies have been made comparing centralized to decentralized appointment systems [3, 4, 5], and they generally recommend a centralized system.

Medical Records

Suggested Placement: Convenient to the central appointment area and to the nonappointment care area. The medical records area can be located on another floor and be connected by a records lift to the central appointment area.

Rationale and Discussion: It should be convenient to obtain a record when a patient checks in at the reception desk. Possibly a record for appointment patients could be pulled at the beginning of the day or even the day before so it is not crucial that records be stored at the reception area although such a placement would facilitate matters for walk-in or emergency patients. Factors to consider when deciding on the location of medical records include:

The quantity of records and methods of recording information

The method used to distribute the records

How the record is received and returned

The role automated data processing will play

Physician Family Care Area

Suggested Placement: Immediately adjacent to the general waiting area.

Rationale and Discussion: A large percentage of clinic users will make only three connections at the clinic: the reception desk, the waiting area, and a family care examination room. The suggested placement will minimize the movement of clinic users [6].

Physician space (examination and consultation rooms) should be made general-purpose/nonspecialized. A central section of shared (overflow) examination rooms has proved very functional, while examination rooms set up for one special use may be underutilized [1]. The doctors should be able to enter and leave the medical space without passing through the public areas.

Ancillary Patient Services

Radiology

Suggested Placement: Near the family care area with separate access from the general waiting area. If the clinic has an emergency room, radiology should be adjacent to the emergency room and should have its own waiting area.

Rationale and Discussion: The suggested placement is predicated on the fact that the link between the accident/emergency department, and the X-ray department is stronger than the link between the family care area and X-ray department. Also, patients may be scheduled for an X-ray without any other appointment.

Other Factors: Setup costs for radiology units are high, and hence many clinics may elect to use contracted services. Data on the use of radiology by specialty [6] indicate that orthopedics, surgery, pediatrics, and general medicine have the highest rates of radiology use. Of course, the expected volume of patients in each specialty must be used to determine the expected volume of radiology used by that specialty.

Laboratory

Suggested Placement: Near the family care area with separate access from the general waiting area. The laboratory could have its own small waiting area or, along with radiology, share a waiting area that includes a single receptionist. Both laboratory and radiology are expensive to relocate and hence should be planned so that each area has sufficient room for expansion.

Rationale and Discussion: There will be referrals to the laboratory from the family care area. A small waiting area is needed to accommodate those who are waiting for a laboratory test. Patients will often leave the lab area and go to the general waiting area for reappointment or billing.

   The cost of a good laboratory setup is high. There are fee-for-service laboratory services available which can be an alternative to a clinic laboratory for expensive tests. One government publication [6] suggests that specimens be taken in examination rooms when possible to minimize patients visits to the laboratory. Their data on the use of laboratory by specialty indicate that antenatal, pediatrics, and general medicine have the highest rates of laboratory use. Thus, if a high patient volume is expected in one or more of these specialties, that specialty should be close to the laboratory.

Physical Therapy

Suggested Placement: It is desirable to have separate access from the general waiting area with provisions for ramp or elevator access for wheelchair patients.

Rationale and Discussion: Patients will wish to make appointments for physical therapy after consultation with their doctor who most often will be an orthopedic specialist. Some patients will be confined to wheelchairs, and this fact should be reflected in the design of the unit.

EKG

Suggested Placement: In many cases, an efficient method of taking electro-cardiograms relies on a portable EKG unit which can be taken to any examination room. If a large demand for EKG is expected, a room for the technician, the equipment, and the records should be provided. This room should have separate access from the general waiting area.

Rationale and Discussion: Consideration should be given to the choice between an EKG unit in a nonspecific examination room and a separate EKG sector with a technician. The choice is mainly a function of expected patterns of use.

The data in one study [6] indicate a large use of EKG by general medicine (17 percent) but little or no use by other specialties. For a separate EKG area, a small waiting room is needed to accommodate those who are waiting for a test. There will be referrals to the EKG area from the family care area. Patients will often leave that area and go for billing or to make a reappointment.

Vision Care

Suggested Placement: Near the general waiting area with a separate access route.

Rationale and Discussion: If the expected demand for services indicates a need for a separate clinic for vision care, it should be near the general waiting area to minimize unnecessary traffic.

Patients may need to wait for a second stage of testing, and if convenient, the general waiting area could be used. If not, a separate waiting area for four to six people should be provided. Refractionists will require a minimum length of 21 ft 6 in. in order to use the direct method of sight testing unless they employ reflective equipment which requires less space [7]. It has been found convenient to place two sight-testing rooms next to each other since each can have a 21 ft 6 in. length and a narrow width.

Mental Health Area

Suggested Placement: Near the general waiting area with a separate access route.

Rationale and Discussion: Placement should minimize unnecessary traffic. The size of this area will depend on the expected demand and on the services offered. A mental health unit may involve the part-time use of two or three examination rooms, and thus make use of the general waiting area and other facilities of the clinic. On the other hand, it could be as large as 7 floors out of 33 and include areas for group therapy, individual conferences, and various testing, rehabilitation, and day care facilities [8]. In the latter case, the unit should include its own waiting areas on each floor. The OEO guidelines [7] suggest that this unit may be located apart from the physician clinic area, but it should have easy access for all patients. However, there may be less stigma attached to a visit if the patients wait in the general waiting area.

Dental Care Area

Suggested Placement: Near the general waiting area and family care area.

Rationale and Discussion: There are advantages, especially for small dental departments, in sharing the use of the appointments and records areas of the clinic. Patients may be referred from the family care area to the dental clinic. If the dental clinic is adjacent to the general waiting area, it avoids the duplication of waiting area facilities. Some clinics have used two dentists in a clinic set up for one dentist by the use of a split 12-hour day as a means of reducing overhead costs.

Surgery Unit

Suggested Placement: Direct connection to radiology and nonappointment care is desirable.

Rationale and Discussion: Radiology is often used in conjunction with surgical procedures. A nonappointment care unit will have cases demanding immediate referral to surgery.

Internal medicine and surgery are logical neighbors because of the close cross consultation between the internist and the surgeon. In locating other activities near a surgical unit, consideration must be given to the necessity of maintaining a standard of surgical cleanliness in these areas.

Nonappointment Care/Urgent Care

Suggested Placement: Near the main entrance with provisions for admitting and controlling patient movement during off-hours operation. A separate waiting room is desirable for urgent care.

Rationale and Discussion: Unscheduled patients may arrive with an ailment causing danger or personal discomfort to other patients. The after-hours area should be near the front door for security reasons, and it should be clearly identified.

The designer must ensure that the after-hours staff will have access to records, laboratory, radiology, supply area, and the pharmacy.

Other Important Considerations

Nonappointment patients (e.g., emergency care) may be disturbing to regular patients. Also there must be provisions for nonappointment evening visits with appropriate safeguards as well as access to medical records.

Other Medical Support Services

These include community area public health, social worker, dietician, public health nurse, etc.

Suggested Placement: The community area should have separate access and should be adjacent to the general waiting area. Depending on demand, a multiple-use office or individual office for support services could be provided with access from the general waiting area. These should be situated such that the access route does not pass the consultation rooms.

Rationale and Dicsussion: Uses of the community area would range from special clinics to health information programs. Since this use often would occur during evening hours, a separate access would facilitate building security. An alternate plan would be to have access from the general waiting area by a corridor which leads only to the community room.

For an efficient layout, it is important to estimate demand for support services and plan accordingly. Since patients may attend a clinic for the use of these services only, a separate access from the general waiting area is desirable. Also, it is desirable not to disturb the physician service area with noise and constant traffic.

Outpatient Pharmacy

Suggested Placement: Adjacent to the general waiting area.

Rationale and Discussion: Patients will visit the pharmacy either immediately after their clinic appointments or as a separate visit to the clinic. In the former case, it is preferable to have them first return to the general waiting area and then go to the pharmacy. Other placements could easily lead to excess traffic through intermediate clinics and create confusion.

Large facilities have found it convenient to have a dispensing pharmacy near the main entrance area [8], and the OEO guidelines [7] suggest enlarging the general waiting area if necessary. In some states, there are strict laws constraining the development of clinic pharmacies. In Massachusetts, for example, the statutes have encouraged the renting of space to a private pharmacist.

Clinic Administration

Suggested Placement: Anywhere convenient to visitors with a separate access route which does not disturb other clinic areas.

Rationale and Discussion: Some patients will need to visit the clinic administration area concerning enrollment, billing, insurance, or other business. There will also be a certain amount of nonpatient traffic to the business office by salespeople, etc. One approach for large clinics is to have separate administrative offices with cashiers and an initial registration area near the main lobby [8].

Plan Administration (for a HMO or Multilocation Facility)

Suggested Placement: In the same area as clinic administration.

Rationale and Discussion: Many of the same records and business machines will be used by both the clinic administration and plan administration. If the plan is too large to be accommodated in one clinic building, a separate location accessible to all plan members is recommended.

General Clinic Services (Housekeeping, etc.)

Suggested Placement: A housekeeping area containing mechanical and storage space and a maintenance shop should be located near a separate entrance. Janitors' closets should be conveniently located.

Rationale and Discussion: Traffic relating to the housekeeping area should not interfere with other clinic functions. A separate entrance for the storage area will facilitate shipping and receiving. It is recommended that one janitor's closet be provided for each floor or 8000-ft^2 area.

General Comments

A facility should be designed with the psychological and cultural background of the user in mind. For example, a tall building may meet with an unfavorable reaction from a suburban community. Also, individuals used to open spaces like mountains, deserts, or large farms may not feel comfortable in very small waiting rooms. It is difficult to quantify cultural and psychological factors, but these difficulties should not discourage planners from trying to incorporate them into their designs. Unfortunately, there is little published information on the cultural and psychological aspects of facility design which can be drawn upon to provide guidance, and planners will have to use their own judgment.

References

1. William R. Shannon, "Architecture for Group Practice: Master Plan by Design," *Group Practice* November 1970, 20-23.

2. Richard Miller et al., *The Health Maintenance Organization Facility Development Handbook* (Rockville, MD.: U.S. Department of Health, Education and Welfare, Bureau of Community Health Services, 1974).

3. R.R.P. Jackson, "Design of an Appointment System," *Operations Research Quarterly* 15 (3):219-24, 1964.

4. A. Soriano, "Comparison of Two Scheduling Systems," *Operations Research* 14:388-98, 1966.

5. Edward J. Rising and John Kaminsky, "Cost Analysis of a Decentralized Appointment System," Department of Industrial Engineering and Operations Research, University of Massachusetts, Amherst, MA., November 1974.

6. Ministry of Health, *Hospital Planning Note #6. Organization & Design of Outpatient Departments* (49-588), Scottish Home & Health Department, Her Majesty's Stationery Office, London, England.

7. *Space Guidelines for Ambulatory Health Centers*, Office of Health Affairs and the Facility Management Branch Procurement Division, OEO, Washington, D.C., November 1972.

8. J. Burgun and I. Ehrlich, "A 33 Story Outpatient Clinic," *Hospitals* 45: 101-105, 1971.

9. U.S. Department of Health, Education, and Welfare, *Planning the Laboratory for the General Hospital*, Public Health Service Publication No. 930-D-10, U.S. Government Printing Office, Washington, D.C., March 1963.

10. Ministry of Health, *Design Guide: Health Centers in Scotland*, Scottish Home and Health Department, Her Majesty's Stationery Office, London, England.

11. Cammock, "Health Centers Handbook," Medical Architecture Research Unit, Department of Architecture, Polytechnic of North London, Holloway, London, England, N78DB.

12. Ministry of Health, *Hospital Building Note #22, Accident and Emergency Department,* Her Majesty's Stationery Office, London, England.

13. Department of Health and Social Security, *Health Centers, A Design Guide,* Welsh Office, Cardiff, Wales.

**Part III:
Planning for Outpatient
Clinic Information
Systems**

Introduction

Chapters 6 and 7 constitute a guide to the design of information systems for freestanding outpatient clinics. Each outpatient clinic (OPC) will have a different information system design that will tend to change over time because of factors such as changes in OPC size, economic conditions, operational objectives, and the services provided. The task of designing an information system can be very complex and should not be undertaken without a thorough study of one's information needs. This is particularly true of computerized information systems which are costly to install and operate.

Since each OPC will have its own unique requirements, this guide will not attempt to provide the manager with detailed, step-by-step instructions on how to design a specific information system. Instead, it will focus on the various issues which should be taken into consideration in designing an information system to best meet one's particular needs. The guide should be useful to managers who must deal with outside consultants or government agencies with regard to the design of an OPC information system. With the help of this guide, the manager should be able to ask the right questions and hence be assured that all the important aspects of the system design are dealt with.

Chapter 6 discusses the concept of information and the ways it must be organized to be of maximum use. One particular framework for organizing information is suggested. With Chapter 6 as background, Chapter 7 presents procedures for assessing the cost and feasibility of manual and computerized information systems. Some advice on implementation is also offered.

The author wishes to acknowledge Eric Kyllonen's major contribution to Chapters 6 and 7.

6

The Organization and Interpretation of Information

Definition and Classification of Information in an Outpatient Clinic

Information can be defined as those data which are perceived to be useful in the decision-making process. Effective decision making is based on the availability of relevant information at the proper time and in the correct form. An information system can be thought of as a set of procedures for the collection, storage, processing, retrieval, and dissemination of information.

Information used in decision making in an outpatient clinic can be divided into four general categories: socio-demo-economic, medical, administrative, and financial. Socio-demo-economic information includes those characteristics which are commonly used to describe the total population in the target area (e.g., age distribution) and also those characteristics which may correlate with some medical items (e.g., sex or race or income as related to epidemiological considerations of certain diseases). Medical information is used for ensuring continuity of services, identifying areas of improvement, ensuring maintenance of standards, justifying and determining the influence of therapies, and providing documentation and a historical record. Administrative information is used in the functions of planning, organizing, and controlling all facets of the operation of the OPC. Financial information relates to cash flows, financial status, costs and rates, reimbursements, grants, and contracts. This section is primarily concerned with administrative and financial (i.e., management) information.

Within each of the above four categories, information can be associated with past, present, or future time periods. Past information forms an historical data base. Present information relates to current events, and information concerning the future is based largely on forecasts and is used to assess the consequences of alternative decisions.

Information can also be classified in terms of the phase of the planning cycle that is being considered: what actually happened, what was planned, and what was budgeted (authorized). Information related to actual events can be expressed in terms of various statistics, accounting figures, etc., while information related to what was planned is based on predictions of future events. Information concerning what was authorized can be used as a standard against which to compare what actually happened.

101

Organization of Information in an OPC Information System

Information must be organized in a manner which will facilitate effective decision making by the OPC manager. The method of organizing information (i.e., in terms of an information system) is called an *information structure*. The main purpose of an information structure is to enable the manager to determine what information is required in the form of reports that are needed for OPC administration, for use within the OPC or for outside parties. First, several factors to consider in the design of an information structure will be discussed, and then an approach to the design of an information structure will be presented.

An information structure for an OPC must be usable for a wide variety of management functions; an OPC manager often must make decisions in many different areas (e.g., supply control, public relations, staffing assignments, etc.). Also, the information structure must allow for the changing information requirements of the OPC manager. For example, the primary concern one day might be with budgeting for the next fiscal year, while on the following day the emphasis could shift to trying to determine the reason for abnormally high costs for a certain program.

Financial information will play an important part in the information structure since money is a common basis for planning, operating, and evaluating various OPC programs. The information structure should reflect some method of measuring the OPC activities in terms of its outputs and resources. Since the concept of a cost center (from cost accounting) is not directly applicable to decisions involving the delivery of health care services in an OPC, some other type of organizational breakdown is necessary. One alternative is the use of the program budgeting concept as described below.

An Approach to the Design of an Information Structure

The following approach to the design of an information structure for an OPC is based on a series of distinct information classifications called *dimensions*, which are relevant to OPCs. Each dimension is used either explicitly or implicitly as an important input in several management activities.

This information structure uses the management tool of program budgeting. The program budgeting concept emphasizes the relationships among an organization's objectives, its programs and activities, the available resources, and their financial representation in terms of a budget [1].

While the following example is a useful method for organizing information in an OPC, it should be recognized that there are other alternatives which may be more suitable for a particular application.

Each dimension is defined below.

Line Items (LI): These are the budget categories used by the health facility. The categories are usually organized in terms of a traditional accounting scheme that is not directly related to the operating activities and objectives of the facility. Salaries, rent, utilities, consumable supplies, and fixed equipment are examples of line items.

Program Element (PE): A program element is simply a way of defining what an OPC actually does. Every OPC has a set of programs which are used to accomplish the OPC's objectives. A program, for example, could be a mental health, family planning, or well-baby clinic. A program element (PE) consists of a specific set of procedures utilized in a given program. A PE is a standardized activity which integrates personnel, services, equipment, and facilities to produce a measurable output from a given input.

For example, a program element might consist of a 2-hour session of physical examinations for elderly people. The PE input would be elderly people. It might use a doctor, nurses, paraprofessionals, laboratory services, examination forms, equipment, and space to produce as a program element output (PEO) a certain number of elderly people who have undergone a physical examination.

Program elements are operated at different levels that are multiples of a unit PE. In the above example, the PE might be operated at a program element level (PEL) of zero, one, two, or three 2-hour sessions per month.

Activities (A): This involves all chores, jobs, or duties performed by personnel who are paid on an hourly basis that are separate from those attributed to specific program elements. Hence, the total time of hourly personnel is completely accounted for by the time devoted to work associated with PEs and activities. Examples of activities would include running errands, attending conferences or classes, and providing transportation.

Services (S): These are optional events which could take place during an individual encounter with the health facility and which are ancillary or supportive to PEs. An *encounter*, as used here, is any contact with a provider where services are rendered. The services are consumed by some, but not all, individuals using a PE. Also, no PE uses the same service for all its outputs since the service would become (by definition) part of the PE. Examples of services would be laboratory tests, X-rays, prescriptions, and consultations. The services may or may not be billable to the user.

Personnel (PS): This is the personnel of the health facility. Personnel can be divided into the categories of salaried or nonhourly (PSNH) and hourly personnel (PSH). To determine the cost of salaried personnel for each salary level, one must know the salary amount (PSNHS) and the quantity (PSNHQ) of people at each level. For the hourly personnel one must know their hourly rate

(PSHR), the quantity of people at that rate (PSHQ), and the number of hours at this rate (PSHH).

Reimbursement Basis (RB): This dimension indolves the sources of funds for paying all or part of the billing for individual encounters with the health facility. These include cash, private or public third-party insurance payments, prepayments, or charity write-offs by the health facility. The amount of reimbursement may depend on the program element and/or services involved.

Funding (FU): This element concerns funds obtained from federal, state, local, or private foundations that are usually designated for specific purposes. The employment of these funds often can be directly related to certain program elements. In addition, the funds may include stipulations on their use with respect to parts of one or more dimensions. For example, a state agency might provide a sum of money subject to the condition that it is to be used only for certain designated program elements. The agency would prohibit its use in certain line-item budget categories (e.g., the money could not be used for advertising or to buy major equipment) and stipulate that certain types of personnel may or may not be employed at certain pay levels.

Space (SP): Space refers to physical locations that are utilized in carrying out the objectives of the health facility. The locations may or may not be directly assignable to one or more parts of a dimension. Certain spaces such as treatment rooms and examining rooms would be directly assignable on the basis of the utilization time by different program elements. Other spaces not directly related to specific program elements are called "overhead" spaces (e.g., the director's office, reception area, etc.) and would have to be apportioned according to some arbitrary basis, such as the percentage of encounters for each program element.

In designing an information system based on this information structure, one must consider information related to the above dimension separately and also in terms of pairs of dimensions. Information pertaining to some single dimensions by themselves (PEO, PEL, and A) and too many pairs of dimensions (for example, A X RB, S X PSHH, etc.) do not seem to be useful, however. A starting point for an information system would be to select the relevant dimensions and pairs of dimensions from Table 6-1. For example, the pair of dimensions PEO X S relates the utilization of services to program outputs and would include information for all possible pairs of values of these two dimensions.

Several methods for classifying information have now been discussed, and design considerations for an information structure were presented along with an outline of a particular information structure. An individual OPC information system may not use all these considerations, and it may combine some of them to create new ones. The general discussion should be used as an introduction

Table 6-1
List of Dimensions and Pairs of Dimensions

FU	Funding
LI	Line Items
PSNHS	Personnel Nonhourly Salary
PSNHQ	Personnel Nonhourly Quantity
PSHR	Personnel Hourly Rate
PSHQ	Personnel Hourly Quantity
PSHH	Personnel Hourly Hours
RB	Reimbursement Basis
PEO × S	Program Element Output × Services
RSHH × PEL	Resources Hourly Hours × Program Element Level
RSHH × A	Resources Hourly Hours × Activities
PEL × SP	Program Element Level × Space
PEO × RB	Program Element Output × Reimbursement Basis
RB × S	Reimbursement Basis × Services
FU × RSNHS	Funding × Resources Nonhourly Salary
FU × RSNHQ	Funding × Resources Nonhourly Quantity
FU × RSHR	Funding × Resources Hourly Rate
FU × RSHO	Funding × Resources Hourly Quantity
FU × RSHH	Funding × Resources Hourly Hours
FU × LI	Funding × Line Items
FU × PEL	Funding × Program Element Level

A sample classification of an OPC subencounter by information structure dimensions is presented below.

Example: Use of special laboratory test equipment for screening of children for disease × during a physical examination funded under a grant from the Department of HEW.

Line Items: Laboratory equipment, laboratory consumables, laboratory, nursing, and pediatric personnel.

Program Elements: Pediatric physcial exams.

Activities: —

Services: Administer, process, interpret, and record results of test.

Resources: 1/10 nurse hour to administer test.
1/5 laboratory technician hour to process.
1/30 pediatrician hour to interpret and record.

Reimbursement Basis: No extra charge.

Funding: HEW grant for laboratory equipment and supplies.

Space: Laboratory (existing space used).

rather than as comprehensive design specifications. What is important is that the OPC manager learn to identify the various uses of a piece of information and recognize how the information can be employed in the decision-making process to best meet his or her own needs. The following sections will discuss the utilization of this structured information in the administration of an OPC and how this and other factors influence the design of an OPC information system.

Information Used in OPC Administration:
Tactical and Strategic

The manager of an OPC is concerned with the efficient utilization of the clinic's resources in order to achieve results in accord with its objectives. The OPC information system enables the manager to determine the interrelationships among the clinic's resources, the demand for services, and the attainment of the OPC's goals, and consequently aids in the decision-making process.

Information used in the decision-making process can be divided into two categories: tactical and strategic. Tactical information is used in making decisions about what the OPC should be doing in the relatively short run as constrained by currently committed and planned resources. It is mainly concerned with what has happened recently and provides the manager with feedback on the status of current OPC activities. Strategic information, on the other hand, is employed in decisions affecting long-term changes in OPC operations, goals, capital acquisitions, and changes in professional personnel. Strategic information can be used, for example, for reviewing the OPC's objectives and selecting strategies to meet those objectives.

By using the concepts of tactical and strategic information, the OPC manager should have a clearer picture of the types of output reports that must be produced by the information system.

Tactical Information

Tactical information is related to the day-to-day operations of an OPC. In terms of the information structure discussed in the last section, tactical information would include almost all information about the specific operations of the OPC.

Encounters and money are two basic units of measure of tactical information. Since the primary purpose of most OPCs is to provide services to individuals through various programs for certain fees, tactical information is often related to specific program elements. An encounter, a visit where services are rendered, is people-based while the money measure is expressed in terms of a cash flow. These two measures and the ratios derived from them (e.g., average charge per encounter in a certain program demand) are the fundamental units of much of the raw tactical information that is recorded by the OPC information system.

The what, when, where, and how of the recording of tactical information in terms of the units of money and encounters can be viewed with respect to various inherent relationships in OPC activities. These include the relation of paper flow to people flow, the relation of information which is required to that which is produced and recorded, the relation between individual and composite information, and the relation between money and time. These factors influence the inclusion of information and the choice of frequency, location, and method of collection of information. Each factor is considered in greater detail in the following paragraphs.

Paper Flow and People Flow. Most tactical information relates to people involved in an encounter. This information is usually recorded on paper which does not flow with the people involved. Since this information often can be recorded at alternative locations and at various times, it is necessary to know what information is generated and available prior to, during, and after an encounter. Certain kinds of information need to flow with the patient and are also required as input to the information system. The alternative routing patterns for the patients also influence the recording of information.

Required versus Produced Information. Information is required for health records, legal records, documentation of utilization, and all uses previously mentioned for an information system. The information which is produced or generated often will not be in the form that is required by certain legal or third-party reports, for example. Hence decisions must be made as to the best method, location, and time for processing the information. Both the cost of processing the information and the frequency that information is needed for tactical uses influence these decisions.

Individual versus Composite Information. Information can be recorded in elemental form as it relates to individuals, or it can be recorded in composite (aggregated) form that does not distinguish among individuals (for example, recording that persons A and B were served by the dental clinic on a given day—individual cases—as opposed to recording that two people were served—composite case). There are advantages and disadvantages to each method.

If the individual information is recorded, then it is possible to relate other pertinent characteristics of the individuals such as age, sex, time since last use, etc. In the composite case, the cost of processing the information is lower, but many of the relationships among information items are not known. Examples of information recorded in elemental and composite form are shown in Table 6-2.

A basic question that must be answered is, What information should be recorded for the individual and the composite cases? It is also necessary to

Table 6-2
Examples of Information in Elemental and Composite Form

Elemental Form		Dental Clinic	Time	Date
Name	Sex	Action	Follow-up Visit Scheduled Y or N	
A	F	Prophylactic	Y	
B	M	Prophylactic	N	
C	F	Prophyl. 1 Filling	N	
D	M	1 Filling	Y	
E	F	2 Fillings	Y	
F	M	Extraction	Y	

Composite Form		Dental Clinic	Time	Date
No. of Individuals Seen		6		
Sex of Individuals Seen	M	3		
	F	3		
Actions Taken	Prophyl.	3		
	Fillings	4		
	Extractions	1		
Follow-up Visits Scheduled		3		

determine the basis of the composite information (i.e., aggregating information by day, week, clinic session, primary health care provider, etc.). Finally, for information relating to an individual, it must be determined whether information is to be recorded separately for each individual (perhaps on a form attached to the medical record) or grouped (for example, recorded on a master form used by a triage nurse or clerk).

Relationship of Money to Time. Information is needed on the cash flow for the OPC, including both expenses and income. By recording information on expenditures for various aspects of OPC operation, comparisons can be made with what was budgeted. In terms of income, the OPC manager (as a result of external forces) may have little control over rates or payments, but should nevertheless be aware of the amounts and timing involved. Time delays in receiving reimbursement under Medicare, Medicaid, etc., could affect decisions on OPC operation.

Strategic Information

Strategic information encompasses a very broad time period—from the beginning of OPC operation to the end of the current planning horizon. It is used to assess the effects of different alternative policies on OPC operations. Strategic information is typically derived from processed and aggregated tactical information.

The strategic information relating to past, present, and future operations serves a variety of different management needs. Information relating to future operations can demonstrate the effect of continuing present policies in the presence of outside influences (for example, the financial effects of a decrease in utilization as a result of the existence of a competing clinic). It also will enable the manager to analyze the implications of a change in the operating level of a program element or a major change in organizational structure (e.g., an OPC becoming a health maintenance organization). Information relating to the present allows for evaluation and comparison with what was desired or intended. Information relating to past operations serves as a basis of comparison with current operations and also for considering the present implications of following alternative policies (e.g., what if certain changes had been made in the fee structure in the past year?).

Strategic information is used to assist the OPC manager in making decisions involving alternative policies which have long-term effects on OPC operations. Since most strategic information is derived from tactical information, a complete, consistent, understandable tactical system is an absolute prerequisite to the implementation of valid, useful strategic information. The user of strategic information must be aware of the ramifications of changes in tactical information inputs (i.e., classification, level of detail, periodicity) on the meaning of the related strategic information.

Some Important Factors Relating to the Design of an Information System

In designing an information system for a particular application, one must make decisions concerning the recording, processing, and uses of information. By giving due consideration to the issues of when and how the necessary information is to be recorded and how it is to be processed and used, many future problems can be avoided. The following paragraphs point out several factors which should be considered during the information system design process. First, several "external" factors relating to the overall system design will be examined, and then the emphasis will be placed on "internal" factors more directly with the mechanics of the system operation.

An exhaustive treatment of the many possible design considerations would be beyond the scope of this book. However, it is hoped that the factors presented will assist OPC managers in making decisions concerning the design of their information systems and also serve as an impetus for conducting a more detailed analysis of their own information system requirements.

External Factors

Extent of Automation. The design of a computerized information system will be different from one where only manual clerical operations are performed. As the volume of information, processing effort, and complexity of an information system increase, an increase in the extent of system automation is usually indicated.

Number of OPC Locations. The number of physical locations that an OPC has is a factor in the complexity of the information system design. With more than one site, the information system should supply the individual needs of each location and also the needs of the OPC operation as a whole. Consideration must be given to the logistics of record and information exchange and the compatibility of identification schemes used for patients, records, and staff.

Population Turnover. The turnover in clients necessitates a policy for dropping users from the active files, such as a removal after a period of inactivity. For each new user not included in the active file, it should be determined whether this person is a previous user who had been dropped because of inactivity and for whom a record therefore already exists. Procedures for enrolling, dropping, reenrolling, and maintaining a count of active users should be established.

Types of Patient Records. In addition to medical information, much additional identifying, financial, administrative, and socio-demo-economic information has to be recorded for each individual. This information could be entered in a separate record for each type of information. In deciding on the number of different types of records to be used, one must consider the tradeoff between the difficulties of accessing specific information on a single comprehensive record and the problem of redundancy with the use of multiple records. Some of the factors involved in this tradeoff would be the length of time required to obtain information from a single-record versus a multiple-record system and the costs of maintaining and utilizing single versus multiple records. In the case of records for members of the same family, there is much redundant information. The common information could be included in one original record for each family, with separate subrecords containing information that varies with the individual.

Specialized Medical Records. A decision that must be made concerning medical records is whether the various specialty areas (dental care, mental health, speech therapy, etc.) should maintain completely separate records for current and historical information or, conversely, combine the information from the different specialty areas to produce some form of integrated record or records. Other factors relating to the information system design are whether or not a problem-oriented medical record will be used and what, if any, cross-reference files will be maintained (e.g., a list of people who have had certain diseases).

Operational Objectives. The operational objectives of the OPC will exert an influence on the design of its information system. Design factors such as the size and complexity of the information system, the type of processing used (manual or automated), and the determination of when, where, and how information is to be recorded, for example, could all be influenced by the OPC's operational objectives. With an objective of significantly expanding the OPC facilities during the first few years of operation, for example, the information system used would tend to be larger and more automated (in order to accommodate this growth) than in the case where the OPC size was expected to remain constant for a long time. Other examples of operational objectives would include minimizing the cost to the patient, emphasis on preventive care, treatment of complete family units, minimizing external referrals, and maximizing the valid use of an expensive piece of equipment.

Privacy and Confidentiality. Considerations of privacy and confidentiality center on the rules for the release of any type of information recorded about an individual. Guidelines should be developed for allowing the patient access to his/her own records and similarly for transporting one's own records both within the OPC and to other facilities. Since each patient is normally assigned a unique identifier, a procedure should be outlined as to whether to use the patient's name or identifier. Also, it must be determined who (and under what circumstances) should have access to the name/identifier cross-reference list.

Security. Security in an information system includes the control of access to areas where raw and processed information is kept and where active and machine records are stored. Attention must also be given to the procedures for the disposal of excess, outdated, or duplicate materials.

Staff Training. An important factor in an effective information system is the proper training of the personnel who operate the system. The training provided should match the level of sophistication of the system. In complex systems, the training of the operating staff should be as broad as possible, covering the different facets of system operation. In this way, the operation of the information system can be continued in the event of the absence or loss of a member of the operating staff.

Internal Factors

Recording of Information. The choice of an initial recording location must be carefully considered for each piece of information. In general, information should be recorded as near as possible to the initial point of generation or access. In addition to determining the location of recording, the responsibility for recording each information item must be clearly defined. The duplication of information requested of the patient during different stages of treatment should be minimized. Those items which are medically significant (e.g., a sensitivity to penicillin) or for which a change in value would be important should be clearly identified on the record.

Flexibility and Growth Potential. The flexibility and growth potential of the information system should be taken into consideration during the initial design stage. The system should be designed to allow for ease of expansion and restructuring. One technique for enhancing the system flexibility is to design the system in terms of relatively independent modules.

Filing Method. The method of filing records must be determined. Filing can be done alphabetically by name or numerically by an identification number. If it is done numerically, the various ordering and visual identification methods should be considered. Procedures should be developed for ordering different materials within the records and also for the addition of new material. Also, a procedure should be established whereby the records are periodically checked for completeness. If a summary sheet is used, the decision must be made as to who will update it and when.

Flagging Systems. A flagging system is used to indicate the status of a patient encounter with the OPC. As a result of an encounter, additional activities may be scheduled. For example, a patient may be scheduled for a follow-up visit, or laboratory work may be required at some outside facility. To ensure that these things are accomplished and that the appropriate actions take place and/or the appropriate results are recorded, a flagging system (or *tickler file*) is used to indicate the next step to take and to denote that the scheduled activities have been completed. This can be done with special lists or forms, separate filing of copies of pertinent forms, putting the record in a separate file, or using some type of indicator or "flag." The method selected should be able to handle three basic types of situations: those which are periodic (i.e., an indication of when the next annual physical is due), those involving a reschedule (i.e., a patient must return to complete a laboratory test), and those which are waiting for results (lab, X-ray, etc.).

Reliability and Redundancy. Some reliability and redundancy should be designed into the information system. Internal checks should be made of the recorded information to ensure that the values are responsible and for cross-checking subtotals. External checks should also be used, such as ensuring that a count of people at some stage of care agrees with the count of individual records at that stage.

The earlier and more frequently checks are made, the sooner errors will be discovered. In implementing the checks, one must consider the tradeoff between improved error detection and the time and expense involved in making the extra checks.

Techniques for Processing and Computation. The processing and computation necessary for each information item to give the desired result should be determined. These techniques include simple and multiple summation, percentages, ratios, averages, comparisons, and differences. For any type of aggregation or computation operation, the procedures should be clearly spelled out.

Retention and Back-up Procedures. Raw and partially processed information should be retained as a back-up for reconstructing processed information in case of loss of results, breakdowns, or errors in processing. The time limit for keeping back-up material must be established along with procedures relating to accessibility and disposal.

Interface with OPC Functions. All OPC management functions that are not interfaced with the information system should be examined to determine whether they can be integrated into the system. Through integration with the information system, an improvement in the OPC operating efficiency should result. For example, it may be possible to integrate certain aspects of bill preparation or laboratory and X-ray order generation into the information recording process for the information system.

Cost Limitations. The cost limitations under which the information system is being designed should be clearly defined. In addition to units of money, the limitations should be expressed in other applicable units such as time, people, materials, and space, etc. There should be detailed assessment of all costs involved (including penalty costs due to incomplete or untimely information) for the system under consideration and also for any alternative designs.

Human-factor Aspects. If adequate attention is not given to the human-factor aspects of the information system design, the performance of the system is likely to deteriorate. It is important that the system be designed so that it can be easily understood by all users. The operating procedures should be clearly stated to minimize the chance of human error. All personnel involved with the system should be provided with an overview of the purposes and functions of the complete system.

Audit Trail. The system should produce an audit trail—that is, all actions must be reproducible and all steps reconstructable. This helps to ensure the consistency of the information system output and is useful in detecting errors.

114

Error Handling. Procedures must be established for error handling, including correction or removal of any entry made and the resulting effects of the changes made.

System Manual. All assumptions, design criteria, and procedures must be included in a design and procedures manual which is made available to all personnel involved with the information system. This manual must be kept up to date with all system changes and additions; otherwise, the system will soon become inconsistent and be ineffective.

Reference

1. D. Novick, *Program Budgeting*, 2d ed. (New York: Holt, Rinehart and Winston, Inc., 1969).

7

A Procedure for Designing an Information System

The purpose of this chapter is to outline an approach to the design of an OPC information system. The proposed design process begins with a determination of the information system outputs based on the information needs of the OPC manager; then it proceeds backward through the system, identifying the specific reports required by the manager and the raw data needed to generate the reports. Once the information system input/output requirements have been determined, the next task is to select the means by which the information is to be processed (i.e., by manual or automated techniques). This is accomplished through cost and feasibility studies of various alternative system designs. The final step involves completing the detailed design of the system.

Information System Input/Output Requirements

In order to design an effective information system, one must begin with a detailed description of what the system must produce as output and what inputs are required to produce this output. In this section, a five-step procedure is presented which will assist the designer in making a detailed analysis of the information system inputs and outputs:

1. Determine the types of decisions which management must make.
2. Identify the information system outputs needed in each decision-making area.
3. Specify the data elements that must be entered into the information system in order to produce the output reports.
4. Determine the source of the input data and the method of data collection.
5. Design the input forms.

Some of the steps in this sequence may have to be repeated several times before a suitable design is obtained. For instance, a certain system output (i.e., report) designated in step 2 may not satisfy a manager's requirements from step 1 or may be difficult to produce because of the lack of data as determined in step 4. The output in step 2 would then be modified one or more times until it did not conflict with any of the other steps. Another possible reason for repeating the design process is that the alternative selected could prove to be too expensive to implement, and a cheaper design might have to be developed.

115

Since the operation of an OPC is ultimately controlled by financial considerations, cost should be an overriding consideration in the decision on an information system design. The number and complexity of the output reports produced will have a direct bearing on the initial investment cost and operating expenses of the information system. Some additional but less important system design criteria include timeliness of the output, adaptability to changes or additions, and comprehensiveness. The issue of cost will be discussed in greater detail in later sections.

In specifying the system outputs, the most important reports should be listed first. The desired output reports should be ranked in order of importance in a "priority list" and then included in the information system design in order of decreasing importance. The incremental costs of adding some of the lower-priority reports may be small if some of the data required by the more essential reports can be reused. By sequentially analyzing the reports in this manner, one should eventually reach the point where the benefits of an additional output report are not justified in terms of the additional cost involved.

Step 1: Determine the Types of Decisions Which the
OPC Management Must Make

The decision-making activities of the OPC management will determine the nature of the information system output. Since the decision-making areas will differ to some extent for each particular OPC, a detailed discussion of these areas will not be presented here. However, some general comments are relevant.

Managers should list all the types of relevant decisions they must make along with frequency with which they must be made. This list is critical because it forms the basis for deciding what information is to be collected and how it is to be displayed. No report should be prepared if it is not possible to state what decision it will influence. Table 7-1 contains an example list for a hypothetical facility.

Step 2: Identify the Information System Outputs Needed
in Each Decision-making Area

The next stage in the design of an information system is to determine what information system outputs, or reports, are necessary to help the manager make decisions in the areas determined in step 1. The term *reports* is used here in a general sense to denote all types of system outputs that are used by management (e.g., lists, special documents, tables, formal reports, etc.). Some examples of types of reports are listed in Appendix 7A.

Table 7-1
List of Potential Decisions

Decision	Frequency
Should an expansion of the facility be undertaken?	Every 2 years
•	
•	
•	
Should an additional physician be hired?	Biyearly
Should a new nurse be hired?	Quarterly
•	
•	
•	
Are fees sufficient?	Quarterly
•	
•	
•	
What taxes must be paid?	Quarterly
•	
•	
•	
Are costs out of control?	Monthly
Staff	
Supplies	
Telephone	
•	
•	
•	

Two basic types of reports are generated by an OPC information system: external and internal. *External reports* are those reports required by state and federal agencies and other outside parties, and often they are not used within the OPC. Examples of this type of report would include reports to the state health department, social security administration, and insurance carriers. *Internal reports* are those designed for use primarily within the OPC. The information content of the reports required by outside parties is usually predetermined by the parties involved, and the OPC management has little control over the report format and frequency. These characteristics are usually clearly specified; consequently, the discussion of report design will emphasize internal reports. The design of internal reports, on the other hand, is dictated by the needs of the OPC management who have the freedom to determine the information content, format, and report frequency.

In order to design an internal report that will effectively assist the manager in making decisions, one must determine the proper information content, format, and report frequency. First, the type and amount of information included in the report should be clearly specified. The amount of information contained in the report should be limited to that required by the OPC manager. With the use of a computerized information system, for example, there is a tendency to produce lengthy reports that contain unnecessary information and which ultimately hinder effective decision making.

After the information content of the report is determined, the format of the report should be considered (e.g., spacing, number of pages, etc.).

The third consideration is the frequency of report generation. The timing of the generation of a report may be based on a periodic need for information (e.g., weekly, monthly, etc.) or an as-needed basis. The frequency with which the report is produced should coincide with the manager's need for the information contained in the report. This may sound like an obvious point, but it is often ignored and managers either have insufficient information or are buried in stacks of computer paper.

After the preliminary design of an internal report has been completed, a sample report should be drawn up (using simulated data where necessary) and given to the appropriate managerial personnel for their evaluation. With the use of sample reports, the manager will be able to judge the value of each report in terms of her/his own expected information needs. The reports should be redesigned, if necessary, so that they fulfill the information needs of the users. This process may have to be repeated several times before a complete set of reports has been designed that contains the proper information without extraneous or repetitious elements.

A convenient method of summarizing the reports to be produced by the information system is to list them in a table along with characteristics such as the recipient(s) of the report, use of report, report frequency, length and number of copies required. In Table 7-2 output reports are listed along the top, and the report characteristics are listed on the left. With the completion of this table for all the output reports and their characteristics, one can do a simple analysis of the information system outputs. For example, one can group reports according to certain common characteristics (e.g., create a listing of all weekly reports or of all reports required by the OPC medical director).

Step 3: Specify the Data Elements That Must Be Entered into the Information System in Order to Produce the Output Reports

For each piece of information that is contained in an output report, there must be one or more corresponding information items entered as input to the

Table 7-2
Table of Report Characteristics

	Reports		
Characteristics	Revenue Report	Number of Physician Visits by Specialty	Etc.
Recipient(s) of report	OPC manager, state or federal government	OPC manager, OPC medical director, state or federal government	
Use of report	Determination of OPC income	Determination of utilization	
Report frequency	Monthly	Weekly	
Length	1 page	2 pages	
Number of copies	4	6	
(Other)			

information system. Once the information content of each report is determined (see step 2), the information items or data elements that must be entered as input to the information system to produce each report should be enumerated.

The data elements associated with each output report can be displayed in tabular form, as shown in Table 7-3. The output reports are listed along the top of the table, and the data elements used in the reports are listed at the left and denoted by E-1, E-2, E-3, etc.

Some of the information or raw data collected in the OPC may be required to undergo aggregation or some type of calculation before being used in an output report. Those data elements which cannot be used correctly and must be "processed" should be identified by placing a "P" in the appropriate space in Table 7-3.

Table 7-3
Reports Versus Data Elements

		Reports		
	Data Element	Revenue Report	Number of Visits by Specialty	Etc.
E-1	Private party payment	x		
E-2	Insurance payments	x		
E-3	State welfare payments	x		
E-4	Medicare payments	x		
E-5	General practitioner visits		x	
E-6	Pediatrician visits		x	
E-7	Dermatologist visits		x	
	etc.			

One possible use of this table is to determine the number of times that each data element is used. Knowing which data elements are in greatest demand (i.e., high number of appearances in the table) could be helpful when one is concerned with how the data elements are to be collected. The table can also be used to detect similarities between the data requirements of various reports with the possible end result of combining two reports that have very similar contents into one report.

With the use of Table 7-2, the frequency requirements of certain data elements can be determined. For example, in order to determine which data elements are required on a weekly basis, the weekly reports would be identified and then the corresponding data elements would be found in Table 7-3.

Step 4: Determine the Source of the Input Data and the Method of Data Collection

After the data elements that are required to produce the reports have been determined, one should then ask how the data are to be collected. In general, the source and method of data collection must be specified along with the OPC staff member who is responsible for obtaining the data.

The possible sources or locations for the collection of data vary with the type of information being considered. In the case of patient-related data, for example, the data sources would include the initial registration process (i.e., data such as name, address, age, etc.), an encounter with a provider at the OPC, and an outside facility.

There are several methods of data collection that can be used. For example, information can be dictated into a tape recorder (e.g., a physician's report), entered on a specialized form, or entered directly into a computerized information system through a terminal.

Again, the use of a table is helpful in summarizing various factors concerning data collection and the type of aggregation or processing required for each data element. Table 7-4 lists the data elements from the previous table along with different attributes of the data elements.

With the use of this table, for example, one can make lists of the data elements that must be collected at various locations. Also, the frequency of collection of data elements can be compared with the frequency of corresponding output reports, to make sure they match.

In designing the data collection procedures, the duplication of input data should be minimized. For example, certain data collected on a patient during the initial registration process (i.e., address, date of birth, etc.) does not have to be collected at each subsequent visit to the OPC.

It is also advisable to use aggregation (e.g., combining weekly figures into monthly figures, etc.) whenever possible to avoid the collection of additional data.

Table 7-4
Data Elements versus Attributes

| | Data Elements | | | |
	Private-party Payment (E−1)	Etc.	Pediatrician Visits (E−6)	Etc.
Attributes				
Location of collection	Billing department		Medical clinic	
Method of collection	Recorded in ledger		Recorded on encounter form	
Person responsible for collection	Filing clerk		Nurse or secretary	
Time of collection (i.e., according to a schedule or as needed)	As payment is received		At visit	
Aggregation required	Monthly summation		Monthly	
Calculations required				
Reports that use this data element	Monthly revenue Patient account		Number of visits by specialty OPC utilization	
(Other)				

Step 5: Design the Input Forms

The input forms or source documents are used to record data in order to create a fixed permanent record and/or to serve as an intermediate step for the future processing or aggregation of the data.

The questions of what documents to use, where they should originate, etc., can be answered with the aid of the data element—attribute table in Table 7-4. By grouping those data elements that are collected at a common location and time, one should be able to design a set of source documents that will satisfy the input data requirements of the information system. The responsibility for entering data on a source document may rest on a single person, or there may be several contributors of data.

As with the output reports, it is helpful to list the proposed input forms in a table along with various characteristics. In Table 7-5 the input forms are listed at the top of the table, and a number of characteristics are listed at the left.

The design of an input form will often require a compromise between the ease of entering the data on the form and the ease of extracting and processing the data. For example, a form that has been designed to facilitate the entry of data by the preparer may be difficult for a keypunch operator to use.

Table 7-5
Input Form Characteristics

Characteristics	Input Forms	
	Pharmacy Request	*Etc.*
Purpose of form	Obtain drugs from OPC pharmacy	
Where/when used	During encounter with physician	
Entries made (data elements)	Patient name, patient ID number, drug name amount, physician's name	
Person(s) responsible for entries	Physician	
Number of copies required	3	
Distribution (where the form and any copies are sent)	Pharmacy, Billing department, Patient records	
(Other)		

The type of processing that the information on the form will undergo will have a bearing on the design of the form. For example, a manual processing method may be used in which the data are read directly from the form by the user, an electromechanical processing system may use an optical scanning technique to read the data from the form, or the data may have to be transferred from the form to punched cards for use in a computerized system. In each of these examples, the input form should be designed to facilitate the extraction of data for the particular mode of processing.

Other considerations in the design of input forms are the number of copies required, form size, and color.

Feasibility Analysis of Information Processing Methods

After the input/output requirements of the information system have been determined in terms of the output reports needed by the OPC management and the data elements used to produce the reports, the next area to consider is the method used to process the information.

Depending on the size of the OPC, the design of the information processing system can range from a completely manual system to a computer system that is owned or leased by the clinic. In this discussion, a *manual system* is defined as any system that requires human intervention at different stages of processing; it might include features such as electronic calculators, reproduction equipment, an automated file system, etc. In situations where the size of the OPC does not justify the expense of an in-house computer but in which a manual system would be inadequate, the use of computer service bureau may supply the needs of the OPC at a reasonable cost.

The number of physicians employed by an OPC (being related to the volume of data that is generated) can be used as a rough indicator of the clinic's information processing requirements. In general, for an OPC with fewer than five physicians, an information system based on an in-house computer would not be economically feasible in view of the current state of computer technology, in particular data entry technology. A manual system should be adequate for most OPCs with under five physicians. For certain aspects of OPC operation involving the routine processing of large amounts of data (as in various accounting and billing procedures), the OPC manager may wish to investigate the use of the computing services of an outside consultant as a supplement to the manual system.

For OPCs with more than about ten to fifteen physicians, only a computerized system would tend to have the necessary information processing capabilities. This is especially true in view of the recent interest in a number of new potential uses for an OPC information system (e.g., medical audit, utilization review, etc.), which indicate a trend toward increased data volumes and more complex system designs. In this case, a feasibility analysis of a manual system would not be necessary. The choice of a system for OPCs consisting of between about five to ten physicians is not clear. In this instance, a feasibility analysis should be conducted to determine the costs and technical capabilities of the various alternatives so that the manager can select the system which is most economical and reliable. In the following sections three information systems will be analyzed: a manual system, an in-house computer, and the use of a service bureau.

When the choice of the best method is not obvious, the value of conducting a feasibility study of alternative information processing methods cannot be overemphasized. Without a detailed analysis, it is easy to underestimate the costs involved (especially for a manual system) and overlook certain technical limitations which may result in future operating difficulties.

Cost and Feasibility Study of a Manual Data Processing System

Knowing the information system input/output requirements enables an OPC manager to make some rough estimates concerning the cost and technical feasibility of employing a manual data processing system. Some of the possible uses of a cost and feasibility study are the following:

To compare the costs of different alternative manual information system designs. The effects of using different input forms, output reports, report frequencies, etc., on the total system cost, for example, can be determined.

To establish a cost figure for a manual system for later comparison with a computerized system. An initial cost comparison between the two systems would be made for a set of the minimum number of output reports that would be necessary for OPC operation. After the basic cost of each system has been calculated, the marginal costs of including additional (desirable, but not essential) reports would then be estimated. The benefits provided by each additional report can then be weighed against the extra (marginal) cost to determine whether it should be used. The marginal costs of the additional reports would be compared for the two systems.

To study the feasibility of producing various reports within specified time limits.

To identify those reports or processing operations which could be done more efficiently using a computer system.

Before starting the following analysis, one should make some projections concerning the size of the clinic's user population and the utilization of the clinic's facilities for the purpose of estimating the yearly volume of input forms and output reports that will be processed by the information system. Since the clinic may grow in size during the first few years of operation, it should be assumed that the clinic being studied is operating at its design capacity (i.e., at the level of its target service population). Estimates should be made of the number of patient visits to each physician over a 1-year period and of the resulting volume of information to be processed. The tables developed earlier should be used for determining the required information system inputs and outputs.

In order to obtain an estimate of the cost of a manual data processing system, it is convenient to break the total cost into three components: labor cost, equipment cost, and facility cost. For each component, an annual cost figure is obtained which is used to determine a total annual cost for a manual system.

Labor Cost: In a manual information system, a very large proportion of the cost of producing an output report can be attributed to the labor cost involved in the collection and processing of information and in report generation. For each output report, the labor costs can be determined from the number of man-hours required to fill out the related input forms and to perform the necessary information processing steps and prepare the report.

Although calculation of the labor cost involved in a report might seem to be a formidable task, the procedure can be simplified by considering the report production as a series of discrete steps and listing them on the work analysis sheet shown in Table 7-6. For most output reports the mechanics of report production can be described in terms of the following general procedures or work elements:

Table 7-6

Sample Work Analysis Sheet

Example: Encounter by type of provider (monthly)

Output Report Title: _____

Step No.	Description	Performed by	Time (man-hours)	Rate, $/hr	Cost	Comments
1.	Handout collect and check encounter form	recpt.	.03	4.	.12	approx 3000/mo
2.	Answer quests. re. encounter form	recpt.	.02	4.00	.08/ ea	approx 3000/mo
3.	Total costs of enc. forms				$600/mo	
4.	Share of above for report				$60/mo	encounter forms have 10 major uses
5.	Collect forms at end of mo.	clerk	.5	3.50	1.75	
6.	Tally provider(s) from each form (3000 forms)	clerk	5.	3.50	17.50	
7.	Make hand draft of report	clerk	1.	3.50	3.50	
8.	Type report & proofread	Sec.	1.	4.00	4.00	
9.	Xerox & distribute	Sec.	.25	4.00	1.00	

Total labor cost	87.75
Annual cost	105.30

1. Completion of one or more input forms
2. Storage of input forms
3. Retrieval of forms
4. Processing of data elements
5. Report preparation

Some reports may require additional intermediate processing steps and/or storage/retrieval activities.

The total labor cost involved in each output report can be determined from the work analysis. The annual cost for each report is obtained by multiplying the individual cost by the yearly frequency.

Several suggested procedures and guidelines for making the work element measurements are given below.

(1) Time measurements (using a stopwatch) or time estimates should be made for each work element. In order to make the procedure as realistic as possible, one should use simulated data corresponding to that which would actually be used in the OPC. The time value assigned to each work element on the work analysis should be the average of several observations (about 10 to 15 should be sufficient) of the performance of the work element. Because of possible variations in the worker's performance of the task, a small number of observations (two or three) may not give an accurate picture of the time involved. Also, since a worker who is knowingly under observation may feel pressured and may not perform in a normal manner, one should allow the worker to become accustomed to the observer's presence before taking measurements.

(2) Refer to the tables in the first section of the chapter to determine which input forms are required for the output report under consideration.

(3) In assigning the time values, an allowance should be made of nonproductive time since a worker will not be able to perform continuously without interruption for any length of time. Factors such as fatigue, delays, and personal needs should be considered when time values are assigned to the various work elements. As a rule of thumb, add a 20 to 30 percent allowance for nonproductive time onto the observed times.

(4) Determine the amount of time needed to fill out each input form using simulated data. This can be done either by a timed observation (using a stopwatch) of the completion of the form by the actual user (e.g., physician, receptionist, nurse, etc.) or by simply estimating the amount of time needed.

(5) Determine the time involved in filing the completed input forms in the appropriate storage locations. As a rough guide, studies of official clerical workers [1] have shown that alphabetical filing typically can be done in the range of about 100 to 200 pieces per hour (including nonproductive time).

(6) The work directly involved with the preparation of a report can be divided into three phases:

(a) The retrieval of necessary source documents or input forms from various files or OPC locations. If possible, the source documents used in producing the simulated output report should be placed in files or locations that will be used during actual clinic operation. The time required to retrieve the necessary forms should be obtained through either a stopwatch measurement or an estimate. As a rough guide, figures obtained for some typical retrieval rates of items in an alphabetical file [1] vary from a low of about 25 to upward of around 150 pieces per hour or more (including nonproductive time). The design of the file system will, of course, influence the retrieval rate. For an extensive file system consisting of several file cabinets, for example, the lower values of around 25 to 50 pieces per hour would usually be more appropriate.

(b) The performance of information processing steps involving sorting, calculations, etc. The tables in the first section of this chapter should be used to determine the processing steps required for each report. Actual time observations or estimates should be made for each processing step.

(c) The final preparation of the report, including typing, making copies, etc. Again, time measurements or estimates should be made of the steps involved.

For a more detailed analysis of how information is collected and processed to produce the required output reports, a flowchart analysis should be used. With a flowchart, one can create a graphic representation of the routes of the system documents as they are processed, demonstrating the interrelationships between the documents and the details of the clerical tasks involved. Since the development of a detailed system flowchart would be a complex and time-consuming procedure, this type of analysis is not recommended for a feasibility study.

A flowchart analysis would be more appropriate in the later stages of system design, after an information system configuration is selected. For example, with the aid of a flowchart, one could produce a detailed description of the system's information flow and procedures to be used as a blueprint for the development of an actual working system or for use in obtaining more accurate cost estimates. For more information on the use of flowcharts, many good references are available [2].

Equipment Cost: Some examples of equipment used in a manual system would include filing cabinets for storage of documents, electronic calculators, typewriters, duplicating machines, and office furniture. Based on an estimate of yearly volume of input forms, output reports, and other documents used in intermediate data processing steps, one can determine the minimum amount of equipment necessary for the operation of the information system. This equipment estimate should be revised, if necessary, as the analysis proceeds.

The yearly cost of each piece of equipment can be determined by converting its initial cost into a series of equal annual amounts, taking into account the prevailing interest rate, or "cost of capital." These amounts are spread out over the estimated service life of the equipment. A widely used basis for estimating the service life of the office equipment, fixtures, machines, and furniture is the 10-year figure suggested by the Internal Revenue Service in its *Depreciation Guidelines and Rules* [3]. Since this figure is only a guideline, a different estimate may be used if one feels it is more accurate. For equipment that is shared with other OPC activities not related to the information system, the pro rata share of usage (designated by F in the formula below) should be determined. The annual cost of a piece of equipment can be calculated from:

$$A = I \times F \times (A/P, i\%, n)$$

where

I = initial cost
F = fraction of total use
n = estimated service life in years
$(A/P, i\%, n)$ = capital recovery factor (crf) for interest rate i and n periods which equals

$$crf = \frac{i(1 + i)^n}{(1 + i)^n - 1}$$

Computed values of the capital recovery factor for various interest rates and time periods are given in tables commonly found in books on accounting and engineering economy [5]. Some values for selected interest rates and time periods are provided in Appendix 7B of this book.

For example, assume that a typewriter is purchased for $800 and has an estimated service life of 10 years. It is expected that only 50 percent of its total use will be devoted to information system work. The cost of capital is 6 percent. The annual cost would therefore be

$A = \$800 \times 0.5(A/P, 6\%, 10)$
$A = \$800 \times 0.5 \times (0.1358)$
$A = \$54.32$

The annual cost should be determined for each piece of equipment and sumed to obtain a total annual equipment cost.

Facility Cost: The annual facility cost is derived from the fraction of the total OPC building space that is directly associated with the information system. The pro rata share of the total facility cost to be allowed to the information system can be obtained from a computation of the floor area that the system will occupy. If a separate section of the OPC (i.e., room, wing, etc.) is devoted entirely to information system activities, the total floor area of the section should be used. In areas where information system activities are included with other functions (e.g., in a reception area), the floor space occupied by each piece of related equipment must be obtained. For desks, file cabinets, reproducing machines, etc., the floor area measurement should include an allowance for clearance and aisle space for the equipment.

The pro rata share of total floor space used for the information system is obtained from this formula:

$$\text{Pro rata share} = \frac{\text{area used by information system}}{\text{total floor area of OPC}}$$

The yearly or amortized cost of the building is calculated by adding the yearly mortgage and tax payments to the interest lost on the funds tied up in any downpayment. Thus, if mortgage and property taxes are $10,000 per year and $50,000 was originally invested in the business, the yearly carrying charge for the business, ignoring the effect of income taxes, is $10,000 + 0.06 × $50,000 = $13,000 if the reasonable estimate of a 6 percent return on funds is assumed.

The total annual cost of floor area for the entire OPC is obtained from the annual cost of the following items:

Building amortization cost = $_____

Utilities (electricity, heat, etc.) = $_____

Maintenance (including repairs, custodial services, supplies, etc.) = $_____

Total annual cost = $_____

The annual facility cost can now be calculated from the product of the pro rata share and total cost:

Facility cost = (pro rata share) × (total cost) = $_____ per year

Total Annual Cost: The total annual cost of the manual information system can now be determined from the sum of the labor, equipment, and facility costs.

Labor $_____

Equipment _____

+ Facility _____

Total annual cost $_____

Feasibility of a Manual System: Other than cost, the most important question concerning a manual system is whether the reports can be produced by their respective deadlines given that there is limited staff available for this purpose. For each report, the time between the last data collection and the due date of the report determines the maximum time available for producing the report. If the amount of time needed to produce the report exceeds this value, then clearly the system will not function. At certain times of the year (e.g., at the end of the quarter or semiannually), several reports may be required. Unless extra personnel are used at this time, the time available for producing each report is reduced.

If the length of time required to produce a report exceeds the time available, either the report content or processing methods have to be changed or a computerized system should be used.

Cost and Feasibility of a Computerized System

OPCs consisting of about five or more physicians generally can profitably make use of some form of computerized information processing through the use of either a service bureau (to be discussed in the next section) or an in-house computer. This section outlines the steps involved in conducting a cost and feasibility study of an in-house computer system in order to help the manager determine whether this would be a viable alternative. By conducting such a study, the manager should be able to ascertain which information system operations can be economically processed on an in-house computer and to obtain an estimate of the total system cost. With that information, comparisons can be made with the manual system and service bureau alternatives.

Since a universal formula for specifying the design of a computerized information system given an OPC's size, data volume, etc., does not exist, this section will not dwell on the technical aspects of computer selection but rather on how to deal effectively with systems analysts and vendors in obtaining designs for computer hardware configurations and system cost estimates.

The first step in the following cost and feasibility analysis is to develop system specifications which describe the functions to be performed by the computer. The next step involves obtaining preliminary proposals that include equipment recommendations and cost figures from a systems analyst and/or computer vendors based on the system specifications. The third step involves evaluating the proposals to determine whether the acquisition of an in-house computer would be technically and economically feasible. This section offers some suggested guidelines for performing each of these steps.

System Specifications: Specifications for a computer system are used to describe exactly what functions the system is expected to perform. The information included in a specifications document usually entails descriptions of the system's inputs and outputs, the computations and processing steps involved, the data files required, and any preferences concerning the type of hardware desired (such as input/output devices). Among the details typically included are data volumes, timing of the input data and output reports, peak volume levels, and the projected growth of the data processing requirements. Since the specifications represent the "blueprints" for the system design, it is important that they be carefully thought out; otherwise they may impose unnecessary restrictions on the system.

In order to allow the systems analyst or computer vendor to develop the most effective system for the lowest cost, it is useful to express the system requirements in terms of essential and desirable features. The features classified as essential (for example, certain output reports, processing times, etc.) would be critical to the operation of the OPC and must be included in the system design. Desirable requirements, on the other hand, would consist of those features which are helpful (e.g., certain statistical reports) but not necessary for the functioning of the OPC. In selecting the essential requirements, one should make sure that they are truly necessary since, as the number of essential requirements increases, the number of possible alternatives for the system design tends to become more restricted.

Although system specifications will vary in form and content depending on the particular application, the principal parts of a typical specification document are as follows.

1. System Inputs (Source Documents)
   Type of documents
   Number of data elements per document
   Frequency of documents by type
   Projected growth in system inputs
2. Information Processing Requirements
   Processing steps required to obtain system outputs
   Input data required for each processing operation
   Data files used in each operation
   Schedule of processing operations
3. System Outputs (reports)
   Types of reports
   Number of data elements per report
   Frequency of reports by type
   Scheduling of reports
   Projected growth in system outputs
4. Data Files
   Types of files
   Number and format of elements in each file
   Procedures for file maintenance and updating
   Projected growth of data files

5. Computer Configuration and System Details

    Preferences for input/output methods (e.g., optical scanning, punched cards, etc.)

    Extent of vendor support required (training, maintenance, programming, etc.)

    Expansion potential (i.e., potential for upgrading to a larger system)

Examples of other items to include in a specifications list would be system cost and limitations on the date of installation. Since pre-specifying an upper limit on cost may influence a vendor to propose a more expensive system than is actually needed, the expression of a cost limit should usually be postponed until the vendor has reviewed the preliminary specifications and has supplied a rough cost estimate. After obtaining the vendor's estimate, one might then include a cost limit in the final version of the specifications list.

Proposal Solicitation: At this point, a set of specifications for a proposed in-house computer system will have been prepared. The OPC manager is now in a position to obtain computer equipment recommendations and corresponding cost estimates from a systems analyst and/or several computer vendors. Usually, the initial specifications are presented to the analyst or vendor(s) for review and discussion whereupon suggestions may be made concerning clarifications or the use of alternative approaches to the system design. A preliminary proposal is then requested which would include equipment suggestions and rough cost estimates. With this information, the manager should be able to compare the system cost and processing capabilities with those provided by a service bureau and a manual system and reach a decision as to whether an in-house computer system could be justified. If the manager concludes that an in-house computer would be a valid alternative, then a final version of the specifications should be submitted to the computer vendors with a request for formal proposals.

If one decides to deal directly with the computer vendors (instead of with a systems analyst or consulting firm), the first step in proposal solicitation involves the selection of a group of computer vendors. In general, at least three vendors should be selected to participate in the proposal process. It is advantageous to use a number of vendors since this will encourage competition among the vendors and provides the OPC with some leverage in negotiating with the selected vendor. Also, the ideas supplied by different vendors may contribute to a better system design. Some factors to consider in deciding which vendors to contact include:

The type of equipment offered by the vendor

The availability of vendor representatives in the OPC's locality

Experiences of other users with the vendor (i.e., what is the vendor's record with respect to equipment reliability and servicing? meeting delivery schedules? etc.)

The level of support for training and programming

The vendor's financial status

After the prospective vendors are selected, and the specifications are informally reviewed with each vendor, and any necessary modifications are made, the final specifications should be incorporated into a "request for proposal" document which outlines the information that the vendor should supply. Since the vendor is likely to have its own particular proposal format, it will be easier to evaluate the different proposals if the OPC supplies a predetermined format which specifies the information to be included about the system. An example of a proposal format is outlined below, showing some typical items that could be included in a proposal. The list is by no means complete—one may want to include other items depending on the circumstances involved.

1. Computer Configuration
   a. Basic computer model recommended
   b. Input/output and storage devices used
   c. Accessory hardware required (e.g., keypunches, magnetic tapes, etc.)
   d. Data on equipment reliability
   e. Availability of equipment for upgrading to a larger system
   f. Availability of maintenance services
   g. Delivery and installation dates
2. Software
   a. Languages used
   b. Availability of software packages
3. Site Preparation
   a. Air-conditioning requirements
   b. Floor space and support needed
   c. Power requirements
4. Installation and Training Assistance
   a. Availability of manuals for installation, programming, and operator training
   b. Training provided by vendor personnel
   c. Availability of on-site engineering test time
5. Costs and Terms of Procurement
   a. Detailed cost breakdown for the individual pieces of equipment in the proposed configuration, assuming it is rented
   b. Cost breakdown assuming the equipment is purchased
   c. Estimates of costs for materials (e.g., magnetic tapes, printer paper, etc.)
   d. Transportation costs of equipment (if not paid by vendor)
   e. Cost and availability of training and maintenance services for rental and purchase alternatives

Along with the above proposal format, a proposal due date and contract award date should be supplied. The due date should allow enough time for the vendor to prepare an adequate response (4 or 5 weeks would not be excessive). By including the contract award date (or estimate thereof), the vendors will be able to quote realistic delivery and installation schedules.

Proposal Evaluation: The process of evaluating computer system proposals supplied by competing vendors basically involves making comprisons of the system designs and costs. The method of system acquisition (e.g., purchasing, renting from the manufacturer, or leasing from a third party) is an important consideration having both technical and economic ramifications. Since the selection of a computer facility that best meets the OPC's needs at the lowest possible cost is a complicated undertaking, this section will present some general guidelines for simplifying the evaluation process. First a method of handling the proposal evaluation process will be outlined, and then the alternative methods of computer acquisition will be examined.

The proposal-evaluation process can be divided into two main phases: preliminary evaluation and detailed evaluation. A preliminary evaluation is used to determine whether each proposal meets minimum requirements and qualifies for further consideration. After the proposals have been received from the vendors, they should be checked to determine if all the information requested in the proposal solicitation has been included in the proposal. If an item is missing or not clearly stated in a proposal, it may be that the vendor misinterpreted some of the system specifications. The vendor should be contacted, in this case, in order to make any necessary corrections. After any omissions or uncertainties have been resolved, the next step is to determine whether the proposals meet the essential requirements that were included in the proposal solicitation. If a vendor does not meet all the essential requirements of the system, the vendor's proposal should be excluded from consideration.

After proposals are obtained from (preferably) at least three vendors that meet the minimum acceptable system requirements, a more detailed evaluation should be conducted. In a detailed evaluation of vendors' proposals, both the system design and cost factors should be considered. *System design* will be broadly defined to include all factors affecting system operation such as equipment characteristics, vendor support, installation date, etc. The cost factors include the initial or "one-time" costs and the continuing costs of the proposed system.

A useful method of comparing the vendors' proposals in the system design area is to list evaluation criteria in a table and note how each vendor satisfies the criteria. Since at this stage all the proposals will have met the minimum or essential system requirements, the extent to which the specified desirable features are included in the designs should also be noted in the table. A similar table should be used for the cost factors, listing the initial and continuing costs for each system. Examples of the two types of tables are given below.

Some typical system design criteria are listed in Table 7-7. This list is by no means complete and is used only to illustrate some of the possible criteria. In listing the design features proposed by each vendor, one should note the extent to which each feature exceeds the minimum or essential requirements.

Similarly, a breakdown of system costs for each vendor can be listed as in Table 7-8. The cost items shown in this table are used as typical examples and are not necessarily all-inclusive. Other cost items may be appropriate for a particular installation. As a general rule, any cost item related to the installation or operation of an in-house computer should be included in this evaluation. In a typical computer installation, the cost of the computer hardware may represent only 25 to 50 percent of the total system cost over a 5-year period. The additional costs incurred are the support costs of the computer configuration and include staff, facility, supplies, training, etc., costs.

After a total one-time cost and total annual cost for each proposed system are calculated, a comparison of the different systems can be made by calculating the present values. Because of the time value of money, the annual costs should be discounted by the prevailing interest rate to obtain the present values as of the installation of the computer. The present values of the annual costs should then be added to the one-time costs to obtain a single cost figure for each

Table 7-7
Comparison of System Designs

Design Criteria	Vendor 1	Vendor 2	Vendor 3
Equipment Characteristics			
Memory capacity			
Input devices			
Output devices			
Expansion potential			
Accessory equipment			
Vendor Support			
Training			
Programming			
Maintenance			
Documentation			
System Performance			
Capability for producing			
Desirable reports (number and type)			
Availability			
Delivery date			
Installation schedule			

Table 7-8
Comparison of System Costs

Cost Item	Vendor 1	Vendor 2	Vendor 3
One-Time or Setup Costs			
1. Site preparation			
Air conditioning			
Power lines and wiring			
Building (renovations, flooring)			
Furniture and fixtures			
Other			
2. System installation			
Transportation			
Testing			
Programming			
Training			
Other			
Total One-time Cost			
Continuing (annual) Costs			
1. System hardware (rental basis)			
2. Personnel (system analysts, operators, etc.)			
3. Maintenance			
4. Overhead (electricity, floor space, etc.)			
5. Supplies (paper, magnetic tapes, etc.)			
6. Insurance			
7. Other			
Total Annual Cost			

system. This technique is illustrated in the following example, which assumes that the equipment is rented. The present value of the annual cost is obtained for the first 5 years of operations.

Total one-time cost $= \$50,000$

Total annual cost $= \$30,000$ per year

Interest rate, i $= 7\%$

Time period, n $= 5$ years

Present value of annual costs $= 30,000 \, (P/A, 7\%, 5)$
$= 30,000 \, (4.1) = \$123,000$

where $(P/A, 7\%, 5)$ is the present-value factor for an interest rate of 7 percent over a 5-year period. In general, the present-value factor can be expressed as:

$$(P/A, i, n) = \frac{(1 + i)n - 1}{i(1 + i)^n}$$

Computed values of the present-value factor for various interest rates and time periods are given in tables commonly found in books on accounting and engineering economy. Some values for selected interest rates and time periods are provided in Appendix 7B of this book.

$$\text{Present cost of system} = 50,000 + 123,000$$

$$= \$173,000$$

Acquisition: There are three basic methods for the acquisition of an in-house computer: purchase, lease, and rental. This section will examine some of the advantages and disadvantages of each method so that the manager will understand the alternatives available and be able to select the best method for his or her own application. Only the general characteristics of each method will be presented here since the exact details of a purchase, lease, or rental plan will depend on the particular vendor.

The first method, purchasing the computer from the manufacturer, is often the most economical in the long run. The computer becomes the property of the user and may still have a substantial resale value after 5 or more years. Also, one has the flexibility of choosing the method of financing the computer in order to obtain the lowest interest rate on a loan. Some disadvantages to the purchase alternative are the risks of technical obsolescence and inadequate capacity to meet the OPC's future needs. Also, maintenance services are not included in the purchase price and must be contracted separately.

Leasing refers to renting equipment from a third party that has acquired the equipment from the manufacturer. Often, the third party assumes a longer life for the equipment than the manufacturer so it can lease the hardware to the user at a lower cost than the manufacturer's rental rate and still make a profit. The main advantage of leasing is the low monthly cost which often includes maintenance services. In a full-payout lease, the monthly rate is applied to the cost of the equipment with ownership transferred to the user after a specified amount has been repaid. Leasing also has certain tax advantages in for-profit outpatient clinics. Some disadvantages of leasing are that third-party leases cannot be prematurely terminated without paying some sort of penalty, there is a lack of flexibility in upgrading the system, and limited programming and consulting services are available from the third-party lessor.

The third method involves renting from the computer manufacturer. The main advantage in renting is the high degree of flexibility involved. The user can select equipment from the manufacturer's entire product line and change or upgrade equipment on short notice without incurring the penalties found in leasing arrangements. Also, the hardware rental arrangement can usually be discontinued without penalty. If the user is uncertain as to what equipment would be most suitable, renting may be the safest method. Another advantage is that full maintenance services are usually included in the rental cost. Renting also avoids the problems of technological obsolescence and affords flexibility should the volume of applications exceed the computer's capacity. The primary disadvantage of renting is that, in the long term, it is usually the most expensive alternative.

The decision to purchase, lease, or rent a computer has both economic and technical aspects. The costs of each alternative over a 5-year period, for example, should be determined and discounted to obtain the present value at the time of acquisition. The advantages and limitations of each method must be considered in terms of the OPC's requirements (for example, the planned rate of expansion).

Once an OPC has decided to acquire a computer through one of the above plans, the next step is to negotiate a contract with the supplier. The contract should clearly state the supplier's commitments to the user, including such items as training, maintenance, documentation, and delivery date.

Cost and Feasibility Considerations of Using a Service Bureau

As mentioned earlier, the use of the computing facilities of a service bureau may be economically advantageous for small to medium-sized OPCs (i.e., up to about eight physicians). As an OPC increases in size above a few physicians, it becomes increasingly difficult and expensive to perform tasks such as billing and statistical reporting using a manual information system. The use of an in-house computer would generally be uneconomical for small OPCs, considering the current state of computer technology. Not only is the computer itself expensive to own or lease, but there are additional costs associated with the rental of space for the computer and extra personnel. With rapid advances in technology, there is also the problem of the equipment becoming obsolete. By using a service bureau, one has the capability of computer processing without the initial high cost and other disadvantages of an in-house computer. If the adoption of computerized processing methods is done initially through the use of a service bureau, one will have the opportunity to test and debug various data processing applications for a relatively small financial investment. As the processing volume grows or as in-house computer systems become more economical, however, it may be desirable to switch to an in-house computer.

The cost and feasibility considerations outlined in this section should help the manager to evaluate the possibility of using a service bureau and enable her or him to deal effectively with a service bureau. It is assumed that the need for computer processing has already been established and that the OPC procedures to be computerized have been identified. This section is concerned with two types of potential service bureau users: (1) the user who requires computer processing but not in sufficient volume to justify an in-house computer, and (2) the user who requires computer processing at a volume which would justify the use of an in-house computer.

In the first case, the user is mainly concerned with how to go about selecting a service bureau that will best meet the information system's requirements. In the second case the user must decide between an in-house computer and a service bureau. This requires a detailed study of the cost of a service bureau versus an in-house computer along with an analysis of the advantages and disadvantages of each. Once an OPC has selected a service bureau over an in-house computer, it should conduct a periodic review based on the considerations discussed below to determine whether the bureau continues to be operationally and economically the better alternative.

We will first examine some of the overall considerations involved in the selection of a service bureau. These considerations apply to both the above types of service bureau users. Then we will discuss some cost and feasibility considerations involved in choosing between a service bureau and an in-house computer.

Selection of a Service Bureau: The steps normally involved in selecting a service bureau are as follows:

1. Determine the information processing requirements
2. Prepare a detailed set of specifications
3. Solicit proposals from prospective service bureaus
4. Evaluate proposals using established criteria
5. Negotiate a contract with the selected bureau

These steps are discussed below, and several possible pitfalls associated with using a service bureau are pointed out.

Step 1: Determine the Information Processing Requirements. A study should be conducted to determine which information system procedures should be computerized. Using the methods of the first section of this chapter to determine the information system input/output requirements and the cost and feasibility study of a manual system as presented earlier, one should be able to identify the areas which require computer processing. Estimates should be made of the volume of data, the number and frequency of reports, and the various time constraints involved.

Step 2: Prepare Detailed Specifications. A detailed set of specifications should be developed in order to define precisely the work required of the service bureau. The exact nature of the specifications will depend on particular application and the extent of the programming performed by the service bureau.

For some applications such as billing and statistical reporting, prepared program packages are often available. If prepared programs are not used, detailed processing steps should be included. Some suggested items to include in a specifications list are:

1. Volume of data elements to be processed
2. Descriptions of files to be produced
3. File updating procedures and expected frequency
4. Description of processing steps
5. Description of output reports desired
6. Time frame of each report (i.e., when report must be received from service bureau)
7. Confidentiality requirements for input data and output reports
8. Anticipated changes in processing requirements as a result of clinic growth.

Step 3: Solicit Proposals. The specifications developed in the last step should be reviewed with the representatives of the selected service bureaus. In making the initial selection of a bureau, one should consider proximity to the OPC and the bureau's past record of performance. Also, other area service bureau users could be contacted for information on their experiences with the prospective bureaus.

Step 4: Evaluate Proposals. The proposals received from the service bureaus should first be carefully reviewed to determine whether they meet the desired specifications. A comparison and ranking of the competing bureaus should then be performed, using certain established criteria. Some of the more important selection criteria to use in evaluating the bureaus are as follows:

Cost: The total monthly or yearly cost should be established. If programs are written, there will be an initial programming cost. Other examples of cost factors are consulting, data conversion (e.g., keypunching the OPC data input forms), and machine-time costs.

Financial Stability: The financial position of the service bureau should be reviewed to determine the bureau's stability. A service bureau that goes bankrupt may seriously affect the functioning of an OPC.

Past Performance: The past reliability of the bureau should be examined. Also, the bureau's experience with other OPCs should be noted.

Ownership of Programs, Records, and Data: The ownership of all programs, records, and data associated with the OPC should be established. Although the ownership of programs by the OPC will result in higher programming costs, there are many long-term advantages. Ownership ensures that if at some later date the OPC decides to switch to another service or acquires a computer, the same program can be used at the new site without incurring reprogramming costs. In addition to owning the programs, the OPC should obtain all necessary documentation and user manuals. It is important that the OPC retain ownership of all records and data used by the service bureau. If the bureau is forced to close for financial or other reasons, there may be problems involved in getting the data back unless ownership by the OPC is specified.

Confidentiality: The OPC input data and resulting reports may contain confidential information. The service bureau should provide assurance that the input and output data will be kept confidential and that access to the data will be limited to only those persons directly involved with the processing operations. For data that are highly confidential, a coding scheme should be used by the OPC.

Protection of Data: The input data and reports should be protected from fire, theft, etc., while being stored at the service bureau.

Error Detection: If the OPC uses programs supplied by the service bureau, there should be some means for checking for invalid input data as a result of keypunching errors, etc.

Step 5: Contract Negotiation. The negotiation of a suitable contract is a very important part of dealing with a service bureau. The contract should state the services that the bureau will provide and the costs involved. The responsibility for data preparation (i.e., keypunching and validation), for example, should be clearly specified. It would be wise to include ownership and penalty clauses for the protection of the OPC. An ownership clause can be used to ensure that all data, files, records, and programs are the property of the OPC. A penalty clause would provide, for example, that a certain amount of work must be done before a payment is made to the bureau and assess a penalty cost to the bureau for work that is not completed within the specified time limits.

Choosing between a Service Bureau and an In-house Computer: When an in-house computer can definitely be justified in view of the volume of data to be processed and the use of a service bureau has not been ruled out, a detailed comparison should be made of the costs, procedures, benefits, and disadvantages of each alternative.

A cost comparison of the two alternatives will often provide sufficient information to determine which would be the better choice. Both a service bureau and an in-house computer (owned or leased) have initial start-up costs and long-term operating costs. The cost factors involved with an in-house computer were discussed earlier in this chapter.

If the comparative costs of a service bureau and an in-house computer are about the same, one should then consider other factors to determine if a service bureau should be selected. Some of the important factors to be considered are summarized in Table 7-9. The main disadvantage of a service bureau is the possibility of becoming locked into its processing methods and time limitations, which could restrict the growth or operating efficiency of the OPC. Also, the total processing cost increases significantly with increasing data volume with a service bureau whereas the incremental cost of increased processing volume on an in-house computer is very small. An important advantage of a service bureau, on the other hand, is that one is not committed to hardware that may become obsolete within a few years as a result of OPC growth or advances in technology.

Information System Detail Design

In the first section of this chapter, the design of an OPC information system was discussed in terms of the required output reports and the corresponding input data. After developing the information system input/output requirements and selecting the method of information processing (see the second section of this chapter), the manager should now be in a position to complete the details of the information system design. The areas to consider in this final stage of system design would generally include hardware selection, information handling and processing, facilities design, system security, and personnel and system documentation. Depending on the type of information processing methods used (i.e., manual or computerized) and the attention given to system details during feasibility studies, some of the detail design work for the above categories may have already been accomplished. The purpose of this section is to outline some of the important considerations involved in developing a detailed system design. These considerations apply (to varying degrees) to all three types of information system configurations that were discussed in the last section.

Table 7-9
Comparison of Service Bureau and In-house Computer

Factor	Service Bureau	In-house Computer
Relative flexibility of processing methods and timing	Low	High
Relative cost of increasing processing volume	High	Low
Additional space required	No	Yes
Personnel required	Usually one full-time coordinator	Operators, systems analyst, administrator (part-time)
Relative control over security of data	Low	High

Hardware

During the detail design phase, final decisions should be made concerning the acquisition of any necessary hardware. These decisions may involve both the selection of the type of equipment and the method of procurement (i.e., purchasing or renting). The actual decisions to be made at this point depend, of course, on the progress made during the feasibility study.

If the proposed information system is a manual one or is based on the use of a service bureau, the task of equipment acquisition (if applicable) is usually not crucial to the total system design. With an in-house computer system, on the other hand, the final selection and procurement terms of the system hardware are major considerations in the system design process. If a specific computer system has not already been selected, evaluations of vendor proposals must be completed at this point in order to proceed with the system design. During this period, negotiations may be conducted with the equipment suppliers to modify the system proposals to the OPC's requirements. Further negotiations may also be required on vendor support provisions and equipment delivery dates.

Information Handling and Processing

The area of information handling and processing concerns the basic procedures used in the collection, storage, retrieval, processing, and distribution of information. During the detail design phase, all information handling and processing procedures should be clearly specified. It is important that formal descriptions of these procedures be developed for even the simplest manual system. For a computerized system, a detail design requires that the necessary programs be written or the processing steps clearly defined in the instance where preexisting programs are employed. In complex systems, it may be helpful to draw flowcharts which illustrate the information flows and operating procedures.

The detailed formats of the forms used to collect input data and of the output reports should be developed at this time if they have not been designed already. This would include both paper forms and the formats for data displayed on a CRT terminal. The input forms and output reports should be examined for consistency in the use of coding and special terminology.

The system design should also include provisions for error detection. Input data, for example, should be subject to some type of validation. In a manual system, validation might be performed with the aid of forms that list the acceptable ranges for the data. For a computer-based system, error detection schemes can be built into the programs.

Facilities Design

At this stage of the information system design, one should have a clear idea of the specific hardware components used by the system and of the requirements for floor space, furniture, etc. The process of facilities design involves consideration of the physical layout of the hardware components and accessory items (e.g., desks, file cabinets, computer, etc.) and the design of environmental aspects such as lighting and air conditioning. In cases where the existing building is inadequate for housing the information system hardware, the facilities design will include plans for the necessary renovations or additions.

System Security

Provisions for system security should be included in the detail design phase. Security, used in a general sense, would involve protection from physical damage (e.g., fire, flood, theft, etc.); protection against unauthorized access to data, files, and system hardware; the maintenance of the confidentiality of data that is sent outside the OPC; and formulation of corrective actions to be taken for any possible malfunction of the system. For example, in a computer-based system where an operator error could accidentally destroy a file, the system design should include the use of back-up files. The designer should study the system operation to identify potential security problems and include remedial procedures.

Personnel

The number and types of personnel required to operate the information system should be determined during the detail design phase. Although tentative estimates concerning personnel may have been made during the feasibility studies, personnel requirements should be reviewed in detail at this time.

In order to determine the personnel requirements, one must first identify the tasks to be performed and estimate the number of employees required for these tasks. It is important to develop job descriptions which indicate the skills and knowledge required for each position. By estimating the work load involved in each position based on estimates of input/output data volumes, equipment operating requirements, anticipated frequencies of processing operations, etc., it is possible to estimate the number of man-hours per year involved in each task. These estimates should include adjustments for time off due to sick leave and vacations.

Another aspect of personnel planning is the training required for the various positions. Provisions should be made for training the various personnel (either within the OPC or at an outside facility) in their respective duties.

For large information systems that utilize several people, an organizational structure should be developed which outlines the supervisory roles of various staff members.

Documentation

During the detail design phase, all system documentation needed to operate and maintain the system should be developed. Since documentation is the physical record of the system design and is often the only tangible product of many aspects of the system design process, it is essential to the effective operation of the information system. The amount and type of documentation required will depend on the particular information system. The documentation needs for a completely manual system where the methods of data storage, transmission, and processing are all visible and easily understood are not as extensive as for a computerized system.

The documentation for an information system generally has three main functions. First, it provides the people who operate the system (e.g., clerks, nurses, computer operators, etc.) with explanations of the various procedures involved. For example, the documentation would contain instructions concerning the completion and routing of the system's input forms. The second function of the documentation is to provide the systems analyst or designer with a detailed "blueprint" for maintaining, modifying, or troubleshooting the system. This section of the documentation would contain descriptions of the flow of information, listings of programs, and schedules for the submission and processing of data. The third function is to supply management with a clear understanding of system outputs and policies for the purposes of administering and evaluating the system.

Examples of some items that could be included in a system documentation manual for an in-house computer system are shown below. The specific documentation for an individual information system would, of course, reflect the system's own particular characteristics and requirements.

1. General Description
   a. System objectives
   b. System definition (terms, codes, etc.)
   c. Output reports and uses
   d. Input documents and uses
   e. List of files and uses
   f. List of programs used
   g. Flowchart of system operation
2. Operating Procedures
   a. Preparation of input documents
   b. Operating instructions for programs
   c. File updating and maintenance procedures
   d. Data validation procedures
   f. Schedules for submission of input data
   g. Schedules for distribution of output reports

     g. Security procedures
     h. Equipment maintenance procedures
     i. Other procedures
3. Detailed Specifications
     a. Program descriptions and listings
     b. File descriptions
     c. Hardware specifications
     d. Descriptions of input/output documents
     e. Other specifications

After completing the detail design phase, a complete description of the proposed information system design should be put into the form of a report and made available to all persons concerned with the information system for their evaluation. It is important that any potential problems be identified and resolved while the system is still in the design stage. Changes made in a system after it has been put into operation can be very costly.

Guidelines for System Implementation

The system implementation process involves taking the "blueprint" produced by the design process and converting it into an operational information system. The major activities associated with the system implementation process generally include personnel selection and training, conversion processes, site preparation, hardware installation and testing, and instituting an evaluation program. Although the implementation phase is not part of the design process per se, it is included in this section because of its importance to the successful operation of the system. Also, there is often some overlap between the detail design phase and the implementation phase. For example, the testing of some parts of the system may occur before the detail design of the information system has been completed. This section will present some suggested guidelines for the implementation of a new information system.

Personnel Selection and Training

One of the largest undertakings in implementing a new information system is the selection of the operating personnel and other support staff and the training of all personnel associated with the system. Since an information system will not operate effectively without capable properly trained people, this aspect is essential to successful system implementation.

The selection and/or training of system operating personnel (e.g., clerks, computer operators, etc.) should be based on well-documented job descriptions (usually developed during the detail design phase). The users of the system—those who contribute input data and who receive the output reports—should also receive appropriate training.

For some information systems (particularly large in-house computer systems), the staffing requirements during the implementation phase will not be the same as during normal operation. During implementation, the need for programmers and data conversion personnel (keypunchers, etc.) may be greater because of the high work loads.

Conversion

Although this book is primarily concerned with the design of a new information system where one did not previously exist, it is also applicable to the design of information systems that are replacements for existing ones. For example, one might want to convert from a manual system to a service bureau or an in-house computer system or from a service bureau to an in-house computer. In order to execute a smooth transition to a new system with a minimum amount of interference to the OPC's operation, careful planning and organization of the conversion tasks are necessary.

Conversion is simply the process of phasing out an old information system and replacing it with a new one. The activities involved in conversion deal mostly with converting files, implementing new procedures, introducing new input forms and output reports, installing new hardware, converting physical facilities, and training the personnel. The proper scheduling of these activities, especially in complex systems, is crucial to the success of the conversion. Program management techniques such as PERT and critical path scheduling [1] are helpful in conducting conversions.

Unless one is dealing with very simple information systems or a conversion to an entirely new system that cannot be compared to the former one, it is usually advisable to conduct a parallel conversion in which the old system is operated along with the new one for a period of time. This method reduces the risks involved in changing over to a new system but has the disadvantage of the expense of operating two systems.

Site Preparation and Hardware Installation

The amount of site preparation required will, of course, depend on the nature of the information system. The physical facilities for an in-house computer installation, for example, may require air conditioning, additional power lines, false floorings, and extra storage space. Site preparation also includes the acquisition of any necessary furniture and fixtures. If hardware (e.g., keypunches, computer components, etc.) is utilized in the system, its delivery and installation should be scheduled to follow any necessary facility modifications.

Testing

Testing is an implementation activity that should be performed before a new information system is put into operation. Tests under both simulated and real conditions are used to predict the performance of the system in actual operation and to detect system errors. Another function of system testing is to provide the users and operators with a period of training.

A few general comments can be made, concerning some methodologies of testing. First, one effective procedure for system testing involves beginning with the smallest units of the system (i.e., manual processing procedures or computer programs) and testing successively larger subsystems until a total system test is performed. In this way, errors at different levels of the system are detected and easily corrected. At the level of a total system test, the system should consequently be free from logic and procedural errors and should be evaluated in terms of meeting the information needs of management. Second, both simulated and real input data should be used to test the system. Simulated data can be used to ascertain the system's reaction to high data volumes, invalid data, and other kinds of error or contingency conditions. The use of real data enables one to test system performance under typical operating conditions. Third, all maintenance and reconstruction procedures such as updating master files, reconstructing damaged files, etc., should be tested. Finally, the test results and any resulting changes to the system should be recorded in the system documentation.

Evaluation

Unlike the testing phase, which is performed before the information system is put into operation, evaluation is the continuing process of monitoring the system's performance once it is operational. Since the amount of testing which can be performed before the start-up of a new system is usually limited by time and economic factors, thorough evaluation is an important part of the system's early operation. Also, in converting to a different system (as in changing from a manual system to a computer—based one), certain deficiencies in data handling procedures or forms/report design, for example, may appear only after lengthy experience with the new system. An evaluation plan stating the types of evaluations to be performed and their time schedules should be prepared before an information system becomes operational.

The evaluation process basically consists of comparing what the system is doing against what it should be doing as expressed in the documentation. Areas to be considered for evaluation purposes are the following:

System timing. Are the schedules for submitting input data and producing output reports being followed?

Machine aspects. Is the hardware reliable? Does it meet performance specifications?

System costs. Are the operating and maintenance costs in line with expectations?

Input forms/output reports. Are the user needs being met?

Training. Have the system personnel received adequate training?

Quality. Are the outputs relatively free from error?

References

1. John Neuner and B.L. Keeling, *Administrative Office Management*, 5th ed. (Cincinnati: South-Western Publishing Co., 1966).

2. J. Eisenberg, *Cost Controls for the Office* (Englewood Cliffs, N.J.: Prentice-Hall, 1968).

3. V. Lazzaro, *Systems and Procedures: A Handbook for Business and Industry* (Englewood Cliffs, N.J.: Prentice-Hall, 1959).

4. N. Barish, *Systems Analysis* (New York: Funk and Wagnalls, 1951).

5. E.L. Grant and W.G. Ireson, *Principles of Engineering Economy*, 5th ed. (New York: Ronald Press Co., 1970).

Appendix 7A:
Some Types of
Output Reports

For an OPC

Encounters by type of provider
Frequency count of diagnoses
Utilization of laboratory tests
Revenue by functional area
Accounts receivable (third-party payors)
Accounts receivable (patients)
Statement of income and expenses
List of common diagnoses
Trends in the above

Additional Reports for an HMO

Membership by age and sex
Membership by benefit package
Utilization rates by age and sex
Utilization rates by type of provider
Hospitalization rates by total membership
Copayment revenues
Trends in the above

Bibliography

Alexander, M.J., *Information Systems Analysis: Theory and Applications* (Kingsport: Kingsport Press, Science Research Associates, 1974).

Awad, Elias M., *Automatic Data Processing: Principles and Procedures*, 2d ed. (Englewood Cliffs, N.J.: Prentice-Hall, Inc., 1970).

Brandon, D.H., *Management Planning for Data Processing* (Princeton, N.J.: Brandon Systems Press, 1970).

Burch, J.G., and Strater, F.R., *Information Systems: Theory and Practice* (Santa Barbara: Hamilton Publishing Co., 1974).

Gaus, C.R., "Information Requirements for Management of New Health Care Organizations," *Medical Care* vol. 11, no. 2, Supplement, March-April 1973, pp. 51-60.

Joslin, E.O., *Computer Selection* (Reading, Mass.: Addison-Wesley, 1968).

Kirk, Frank G., *Total System Development for Information Systems* (New York: John Wiley & Sons, 1973).

Levey, S., and Loomba, N.P., *Health Care Administration: A Managerial Perspective* (Philadelphia: J.B. Lippincott Co., 1973).

Li, David H., *Design and Management of Information Systems* (Science Research Associates, Inc., 1972).

Moder, J., and Philips, C.R., *Project Management with Pert and CPM*, 2d ed. (New York: Van Nostrand Reinhold, 1970).

Sharpe, William F., *The Economics of Computers* (New York: Columbia University Press, 1969).

Solomon, I.I., and Weingart, L.O., *Management Uses of the Computer* (New York: Harper and Row, 1966).

Walker, D.E. (ed.), *Information System Science and Technology*, Third Congress on Information System Science and Technology (Washington: Thompson Book Co., 1967).

Harvard Center for Community Health and Medical Care, *Information Needs, Information Systems: Some Concerns for Developing HMO's Reflecting the Experiences of Eight Operational Plans,* July 1975.

U.S. Dept. of HEW, *Guidelines for Producing Uniform Data for Health Care Plans*, DHEW Publication No. (HSM) 73-3005, July 1972.

Index

Index

Accessibility of facilities, 11, 25
Additions to facility, 8-9
Administration, placement of services, 94
Appointment and communication area, 88
Architect, 49-50, 67, 68-71
Attractiveness function, 27-28
Audit trail, 113

Back-up information systems, 113
Bubble design, 68-70, 79

Census data, 15, 23-24
Community participation, 9, 13, 21
Computer information systems, 118, 122, 123, 130-142; costs, 134-137; method of acquisition, 137-138; service bureau, 138-142
Computer model for location planning, 25-40
Construction of facilities, 8, 52-53, 73
Costs, community, 37; construction, 8, 73; fixed, 34-38; operating, 34-38; information system, 115-116, 124-129, 134-137, 138

Demand for services, 16, 17, 26, 27-34, 50, 75-77
Dental care facilities, 65-66, 92
Design committee, 49, 67-71
Design of facilities. *See* Layout of ambulatory care facilities
Distance, effects on utilization and choice, 5-6, 9-10, 17-18, 27, 29-30

EKG, 90-91
Emergency care. *See* Urgent care
Equipment cost for manual information system, 127-128
Examination rooms, 58-65, 70, 89

Facility cost for manual information system, 128-129

Filing methods, 112
Financial information, 102-106
Flagging systems, 112

Geographic potential, 18-19, 20

Health maintenance organizations, 6, 9-10, 27, 151
Health Systems Agencies, 8, 13, 14, 15, 23, 25

Information systems, 99-149; computerized, 110, 118, 122, 123, 130-142; conversion, 147; costs of, 115-116, 124-129, 134-137, 138; design detail, 142-146; external factors related to design, 110-111; evaluation, 148-149; installation, 147; internal factors related to design, 111-114; manual, 110, 122-130; personnel needed, 144, 146-147; reports, 117-118; requirements of, 115; testing, 148
Input of information systems, 115, 120-122

Labor cost for manual information system, 124-127
Laboratory facilities, 65, 90-91
Layout of ambulatory care facilities, 49-95
Land, purchase of, 71
Load on areas in facility, 55
Location of ambulatory care facilities, 3-45
Loyalty factor, 18-19

Manual information systems, 122-130, 143; feasibility of, 130; total annual cost, 129
Master plan, 49
Medical records, in information systems, 110; placement of area, 88-89
Medicare and Medicaid, 17

About the Author

Richard J. Giglio is a professor of industrial engineering and operations research and an adjunct professor of public health at the University of Massachusetts. He received the B.S. from Massachusetts Institute of Technology and the M.S. and Ph.D. from Stanford University.

Dr. Giglio has published and consulted extensively in operations research and systems analysis applied in a variety of fields with emphasis on capital investment planning and scheduling. His work on health systems has focused on ambulatory care and he has been a consultant to planning agencies, health facilities, and the World Health Organization.